Suffering and Spirituality

The Path to Illness Healing

by

Lorraine M. Wright, RN, PhD

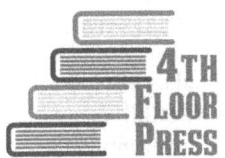

www.4thfloorpress.com

Copyright © 2017 Lorraine M. Wright

ALL RIGHTS RESERVED. NO PART OF THIS PUBLICATION MAY BE REPRODUCED IN ANY FORM OR BY ANY MEANS WITHOUT THE EXPRESS PRIOR WRITTEN CONSENT OF THE PUBLISHER AND/OR AUTHOR.

Suffering and Spirituality: The Path to Illness Healing is an expression of the Author's opinions, knowledge, insights, and beliefs based on her clinical research, clinical practice, and personal experience. Due to the sensitive nature of the clinical and personal narratives, some names have been changed to protect the identities of those involved.

Library and Archives Canada Cataloguing in Publication

Wright, Lorraine M., 1944-
[Spirituality, suffering, and illness]
Suffering and spirituality : the path to illness healing / by Lorraine M. Wright, RN, PhD. -- Revised edition.

Revision of: Spirituality, suffering, and illness.
Includes bibliographical references and index.
Issued in print and electronic formats.

ISBN 978-1-897530-85-6 (softcover).
ISBN 978-1-897530-86-3 (Kindle).
ISBN 978-1-897530-87-0 (EPUB)

1. Nurse and patient. 2. Suffering. 3. Spirituality. 4. Nursing. 5. Palliative treatment. I. Title. II. Title: Spirituality, suffering, and illness

RT86.3.W75 2017   610.7306'99   C2017-900633-9
C2017-900634-7

Published by 4th Floor Press, Inc.
www.4thfloorpress.com
1st Printing 2017
Printed in Canada
Cover Image from istockphoto.com

DEDICATION

To the loving memory of my amazing parents,
Hazel Jean Schollar Wright and James William Wright,
and my dear, wise friend of fifty years,
Thelma Midori Kosaka, who are with me always.

In the rising sun and its going down,
we remember them.
In the blowing of the wind and in the chill of winter,
we remember them.
In the opening of buds and in the rebirth of spring,
we remember them.
In the rustling of leaves and in the beauty of autumn,
we remember them.
In the beginning of the year and when it ends,
we remember them.
When we are weary and in need of strength,
we remember them.
When we are lost and sick at heart,
we remember them.
When we have joys we wish to share,
we remember them.
So as long as we live, they too shall live,
For they are now a part of us,
as we remember them.

Memorial Prayers, Rabbi's Manual
General Conference of American Rabbis

TABLE OF CONTENTS

OTHER BOOKS	VI
EDUCATIONAL DVDS	VII
ACKNOWLEDGMENTS	IX
INTRODUCTION	1
CHAPTER 1: Suffering and Spirituality in Everyday Life	13
CHAPTER 2: Suffering and Illness	29
CHAPTER 3: Spirituality and Illness	83
CHAPTER 4: The Trinity Model: Beliefs, Suffering, and Spirituality	123
CHAPTER 5: Spiritual Care Practices	158
CHAPTER 6: Connecting the Personal and the Professional	227
MOVIES	240
ABOUT THE AUTHOR	244
AUTHOR CONTACT INFORMATION	246
INDEX	247

OTHER BOOKS BY
LORRAINE M. WRIGHT

Wright, L.M. (2013). *Don't get married….unless.* Calgary, AB: 4th Floor Press.

Wright, L.M., & Leahey, M. (2013). *Nurses and families: A guide to family assessment and intervention* (6th ed.). Philadelphia, PA: F.A. Davis. (Previous editions: 1st ed. 1984; 2nd ed. 1994; 3rd ed. 2000; 4th ed. 2005; 5th ed. 2009). Translations in French, German, Icelandic, Portuguese, Japanese, Spanish and Swedish.

Wright, L.M., & Bell, J.M. (2009). *Beliefs and illness: A model for healing.* Calgary, AB: 4th Floor Press. Translation in Japanese.

Wright, L.M. (2005). *Spirituality, suffering, and illness: Ideas for healing.* Philadelphia, PA: F.A. Davis. Translations in Portuguese and Japanese.

Wright, L.M., Watson, W.L., & Bell, J.M. (1996). *Beliefs: The heart of healing in families and illness.* New York, NY: Basic Books. Translations in Japanese and Swedish.

Bell, J.M., Watson, L.W., & Wright, L.M. (Eds.). (1990). *The cutting edge of family nursing.* Calgary, AB: Family Nursing Unit Publications.

Bell, J.M., Wright, L.M., Leahey, M., Watson, W.L., & Chenger, P.L. (Eds.). (1988). *International family nursing conference proceedings.* University of Calgary, Calgary, AB.

Leahey, M., & Wright, L.M. (Eds.). (1987). *Families and life-threatening illness.* Springhouse, PA: Springhouse.

Leahey, M., & Wright, L.M. (Eds.). (1987). *Families and psychosocial problems.* Springhouse, PA: Springhouse.

Wright, L.M., & Leahey, M. (Eds.). (1987). *Families and chronic illness.* Springhouse, PA: Springhouse.

Educational DVDs by Lorraine M. Wright

Wright, L.M. (Producer). (2016). *Therapeutic Conversations with Families: What's love got to do with it?* [DVD]. (Available from: www.lorrainewright.com/lovedvd.htm)

Wright, L.M. [Producer]. (2007). *Spirituality, Suffering, and Illness: Conversations for healing.* [DVD]. (Available from: www.lorrainewright.com/sufferingdvd.htm)

Wright, L.M. & Leahey, M. (Producers). (2010). *Common errors in family interviewing: How to avoid and correct.* [DVD]. (Available from: www.FamilyNursingResources.com)

Wright, L.M. & Leahey, M. (Producers). (2010). *How to interview Families of the Elderly: Tips and Microskills.* [DVD]. (Available from: www.FamilyNursingResources.com)

Wright, L.M. & Leahey, M. (Producers). (2010). *How to interview an Individual to Gain a Family Perspective: A clinical demonstration.* [DVD]. (Available from: www.FamilyNursingResources.com)

Wright, L.M. & Leahey, M. (Producers). (2006). *How to use questions in family interviewing.* [DVD]. (Available from: www.FamilyNursingResources.com)

Wright, L.M. & Leahey, M. (Producers). (2003). *How to intervene with families with health concerns.* [DVD]. (Available from: www.FamilyNursingResources.com)

Wright, L.M. & Leahey, M. (Producers). (2002). *Family Nursing Interviewing Skills: How to engage, assess, intervene, and terminate.* [DVD]. (Available from: www.FamilyNursingResources.com)

Wright, L.M. & Leahey, M. (Producers). (2001). *Calgary Family Assessment Model: How to apply in clinical practice.* [DVD]. (Available from: www.FamilyNursingResources.com)

Wright, L.M. & Leahey, M. (Producers). (2000). *How to do a 15 minute (or less) family interview.* [DVD]. (Available from: www.FamilyNursingResources.com)

ACKNOWLEDGMENTS

Special thanks and appreciation to:

• Anne Bougie-Johnson, President, 4th Floor Press, Inc. and Literary Agent, Sparks Literary Consultants Inc., Calgary, Canada for your willingness to shepherd yet another manuscript of mine from initial draft through to publication. Your critique and suggestions are always well conceptualized, thoughtful, and informative. Your encouragement, wisdom, humor, and cheerleading throughout the writing/research process kept me motivated and believing in the future contribution of this 2nd edition.

• Karen Georghiou, Anne Bougie-Johnson, and my late dear friend Thelma Midori Kosaka who graciously and generously accepted my invitation to share their suffering and spirituality reflections within the context of their illness narratives. Your contributions were poignant, reflective, and heartfelt. I learned from and was inspired by each of you.

• Debbie McLeod, RN, PhD, for your permission to use parts of your excellent chapter from the first edition of this book.

• Juliet Thornton, RN, MN, who was one of the clinicians of a family described in this text, and who gave so much of her knowledge, compassion, and herself.

• The individuals, couples and families in my

own independent practice; the families with whom I have been honored to meet and interview in various countries worldwide; as well as the couples/families within the outpatient clinic of the Family Nursing Unit, University of Calgary. I have been privileged to learn from and assist families in softening their suffering for some forty-plus years! Their illness stories of suffering, hope, and healing have taught and transformed me as a clinician, a nurse educator, and a woman. The collection of illness stories that I carry within me has profoundly softened my heart and touched my spirit.

Lorraine M Wright

March, 2017

INTRODUCTION

Sickness and trouble and worry and love,
these things will mess with you at every level of life.
Domhnall Gleeson

Have you escaped suffering in your life? Do you know anyone who has shunned suffering? Usually, anyone who breathes experiences suffering, some more, some less. Over time, we learn that part of being human is to suffer. For many of us, the first time we experienced deep suffering was our first heartbreak in a relationship or the first death of a loved one or pet. This is often our initial realization that deep love and deep suffering are the same. Serious illness and/or disability can also invite deep suffering when our lives and relationships are changed forever by these experiences. But, suffering does not occur in a vacuum. I have learned from both personal and professional experiences that deep suffering opens the door to spirituality as attempts are made to make sense of and to heal from suffering. Suffering and spirituality are an inseparable duo.

Suffering and Spirituality: The Path to Illness Healing aims to contribute to our understanding of the influence and power of suffering and spirituality on the path to hope and illness healing. It offers healthcare professionals particular spiritual care practices that have the possibility of facilitating healing for those experiencing serious illness, loss, and/or disability. This is *not* a book about various religious traditions and health, although a knowledge of various faith traditions of course can add appreciation to how clients/families respond to illness.

To my knowledge, this revised edition remains the only text for healthcare professionals that acknowledges the inter-relationship between suffering and spirituality and provides a comprehensive discussion of the importance of these concepts within the context of illness. It also emphasizes the impact and influence of the family when serious illness arises, rather than simply focusing on the individual. The connection between suffering and spirituality is perhaps best illuminated through actual clinical examples of persons/families experiencing illness that are sprinkled generously throughout this text.

Healthcare professionals frequently encounter patients/families who are experiencing deep suffering. It is essential that we are prepared to respond with spiritual sensitivity to clients and family members who have or are experiencing serious illness, death, addiction, abuse, loss, environmental, war, or terrorist catastrophes and to learn what kinds of therapeutic conversations and spiritual practices can best assist or inhibit hope and healing.

SUFFERING AND SPIRITUALITY IN THE CONTEXT OF ILLNESS

Healthcare professionals form relationships with individuals, families, and communities to promote health and "soften suffering." I am grateful to Marga Thome, University of Iceland (personal communication, June 6, 2006) for offering me the meaningful phrase of "softening suffering" to describe lessening the intensity of suffering. She suggested this phrase "soften suffering" while I was presenting a workshop in Iceland entitled Spirituality, Suffering, and Illness. This term resonated with me and fit my professional/personal experiences rather than the use of the terms "diminish," "alleviate," or "reduce" suffering as I had suggested in the first edition of this book (Wright, 2005). Those terms suggest that suffering can somehow be measured, but, of course, this painful human phenomenon cannot be calculated. In this revised edition, the preferred phrase to describe the core of my clinical work with families is to "soften suffering."

Indeed, I believe that the very heart of most healthcare professionals' practice is the encounter with suffering. Traditionally, many healthcare professions have professed to apply holistic approaches to caring for others and themselves, and offered interventions that incorporate the biopsychosocial-spiritual domains of life. However, the spiritual domain has often been neglected, overlooked, or forgotten by healthcare professionals. But, spirituality has been found to play a key role in one's health and illness. Illness suffering leads one into the spiritual domain of life.

In this text, the term "spirituality" designates the human desire for a sense of meaning, purpose, connection, and fulfillment through intimate relationships and life experiences. It is the essence of who we are as humans. When serious illness arises in the life of an individual, it is often accompanied by suffering as one attempts to make sense (or not) of this frequently life altering experience. An experience of illness suffering leads one into the spiritual domain and invites questions about the big issues in life such as: Why do I have this serious illness? How will my family cope? What did I do to deserve this illness?-Why is this happening to me? What am I supposed to learn from this suffering?

Suffering and Spirituality: The Path to Illness Healing provides a framework of knowledge, values, skills, and experiences for healthcare professionals seeking to understand the connection between suffering and spirituality. It explores and examines the role of spirituality in suffering and healing and vice versa. Readers are given an opportunity to participate in an open and critical reflection on the spiritual experiences of patients, caregivers, other healthcare professionals, and themselves. In addition, they are invited to reflect on their own spirituality and how it may impact their healthcare and relationships with others.

SOME BACKGROUND AND EVOLUTION OF THINKING AND CLINICAL RESEARCH

This book was the next logical progression in my theoretical, research, and clinical practice ideas for assisting individuals and families who are experiencing deep suffering. FA Davis Company has supported my ideas by publishing six editions of my co-authored book with Dr. Maureen Leahey entitled *Nurses and Families: A Guide to Family Assessment and Intervention* (2013). In that text for generalist practice for nurses working with families, we have a sub-category called 'Religion and Spirituality' within the Calgary Family Assessment Model. The 'Nurses and Families' text gives a brief description and definition of spirituality and religion and a few examples of questions that could be asked of a family. However, it is very limited in its discussion about this topic as that was not the focus of that particular text.

In 1996, Drs. Wendy L. Watson, Janice M. Bell, and I co-authored a book entitled *Beliefs: The Heart of Healing in Families and Illness* published by Basic Books, New York. From our clinical research, we became more convinced that what families believe about their illness experience is the most significant influence on how they cope with their illness. Therefore, in our 'Beliefs' text, we dramatically expanded our ideas, knowledge, and understanding of beliefs. This learning was primarily gained through a research project that culminated in the writing of that text and in the development of the Illness Beliefs Model for advanced practice for healthcare professionals.

In 2009, Dr. Janice Bell and I published a major revision and update of the original 'Beliefs' text with new research and clinical examples. The text was also given a revised title of *Beliefs and Illness: A Model for Healing*. We encourage clinicians to explore a variety of beliefs about the illness experience. For example, we promote exploration of beliefs about etiology, diagnosis, prognosis, role of family members and healthcare professionals, and spirituality/religion. I mention my previous co-authored texts because this current text has been a natural flow from these previous books.

Beliefs and Illness: A Model for Healing was clearly focused on the beliefs of patients, families, and healthcare professionals about illness. But, in this *Suffering and Spirituality* text, I emphasize the interconnection between illness beliefs, suffering, and spirituality.

For the past twenty-plus years, I have been developing my theoretical ideas, definitions, and descriptions of the concepts of suffering and spirituality. In my clinical practice and in previous supervision of my graduate nursing students' clinical practice, I have been examining conversations of suffering and spirituality with persons experiencing serious illness. Over the years, I have increased my publishing and presentations of these ideas about suffering and spirituality in the context of illness. I also developed and taught the first course of Spirituality in Health and Illness in the Faculty of Nursing, University of Calgary. In addition, I wrote and produced an educational DVD entitled *Spirituality, Suffering, and Illness: Conversations for Healing* where I discussed the theory and demonstrated an actual interview with a family (Wright, 2007).

It has now been twelve years since the first edition of this book and my thinking about suffering and spirituality has expanded even further. One of the most influential aspects to my current thinking and spiritual care practices has been the great privilege of travelling and lecturing worldwide. My learning about illness suffering and spiritual care practices in various countries has been enhanced by conducting family interviews not only in various places within my own country of Canada, but also in Brazil, Denmark, Iceland, Indonesia, Japan, Qatar, Switzerland, Thailand, and United States. Suffering is a universal phenomenon! Spiritual care practices that have a foundation of love and compassion enable illness suffering to be softened, and hope and healing to begin. To demonstrate the spiritual care practice that brings forth the healing power of love, I wrote/produced an educational DVD entitled *Therapeutic Conversations with Families: What's Love Got to Do with It?* (Wright, 2016).

UNIQUENESS OF THIS TEXT

Other professional texts have focused on **either** suffering **or** spirituality and/or religion. The main distinguishing feature that differentiates this book from others is twofold: 1. This revised edition still remains the only textbook for healthcare professionals that connects suffering and spirituality in a meaningful and thought-provoking manner. In some texts on spirituality, the word suffering is not even listed in the index. 2. This text continues to have thick and rich descriptions of actual clinical work with ideas for specific spiritual care practices that can be utilized to soften suffering within the context of illness. Descriptions of research-based practice and practice-based research are a meaningful component of this book.

A TOUR OF THE CHAPTERS

This book is conceptualized in three different parts. This first part is to invite the reader to consider notions and experiences of spirituality and suffering within the context of illness. Afterward, the reader is gently brought from that reflection to specific discussions of the concepts of suffering and spirituality as the pathway to healing. Finally, the third part is to connect these two concepts of suffering and spirituality and to apply them in clinical practice through the rich sprinkling of clinical examples. These clinical examples will be the guideposts for how healthcare professionals can bring forth conversations of suffering and spirituality that have the potential for healing when working with individuals/families.

Chapter 1 invites the reader to reflections about what is considered suffering and spirituality within the context of illness through various stories. These illness stories offer insights as to how suffering and spiritual beliefs and practices play out in interactions between patients/families and healthcare providers.

Chapter 2 offers highlights from my learnings and reflections about illness suffering and how it affects health and illness responses. This brings the reader into the current notions and broad range of opinions about what is suffering with clinical examples.

Chapter 3 offers descriptions of spirituality and its relationship to health and illness. Useful distinctions are made between spirituality and religion. It also offers a caution to not objectify spirituality in clinical practice.

Chapter 4 offers a conceptual model, namely, the Trinity Model, as a way of understanding the inter-connectedness between beliefs, suffering, and spirituality. Two clinical examples are offered that beautifully illustrate this model and its trinity of concepts and how they may be observed and acknowledged in clinical practice.

Chapter 5 presents the spiritual care practices that are necessary for softening suffering from illness, loss, and/or disability. The key ingredients for such practices include: engaging suffering strangers; acknowledging suffering and the sufferer; bringing forth suffering markers; telling, listening to, and witnessing suffering; creating a healing context; inviting reflections about illness suffering; reverencing, loving and compassionate relationship between a clinician and patient/family; and challenging constraining beliefs about illness suffering. Several clinical vignettes are offered to invite a vision of this type of practice.

Chapter 6 calls for healthcare professionals to connect their personal and professional lives in order to provide more genuine therapeutic conversations with their clients. Of course, the final chapter would not be complete without the final word being comments and statements from both healthcare professionals and patients/families about how their lives and relationships are changed when conversations of suffering and spirituality in the midst of serious illness are invited to be spoken.

MY HOPE FOR THIS BOOK

My sincere hope is that this book will provide healthcare professionals with a thorough and comprehensive understanding of the interconnectedness of beliefs, suffering, and spirituality within an illness context. Therefore, I offer a particular conceptual model, namely the Trinity Model (see Chapter 4), to enable and encourage healthcare professionals to bring forth conversations of illness beliefs, suffering, and spirituality in clinical practice with ill persons and their family members. By knowing how to bring these conversations forth and what questions to ask, we can invite healing and soften suffering.

The influence of family members' spiritual and religious beliefs on their illness experiences has been one of the most neglected areas in healthcare, despite some professional origins, particularly nursing, which have a strong historical religious base. However, there is evidence that healthcare professionals are waking up to this neglected aspect in clinical practice. Increasing numbers of articles in professional journals and a handful of books with an emphasis on spirituality are now available. This revised edition, ***Suffering and Spirituality: The Path to Illness Healing***, adds to that body of knowledge. But, an important contribution is the offering of very specific ideas of "how to" engage individuals and families in conversations about suffering and spirituality that have the potential to invite illness healing. I trust that this book can be a meaningful touchstone to provide the kind of compassionate care that healthcare professionals are capable of providing and that ill persons and their families are eager to receive.

REFERENCES

Wright, L.M. [Producer]. (2007). *Spirituality, suffering, and illness: converstations for healing. [DVD].* (Available from: www.lorrainewright.com/sufferingdvd.htm)

Wright, L.M. (2005). *Spirituality, suffering, and illness: Ideas for healing.* Philadelphia: FA Davis Co.

Wright, L.M. (Producer). (2016). *Therapeutic Conversations with Families: What's love got to do with it?* [DVD]. (Available from: www.lorrainewright.com/lovedvd.htm)

Wright, L.M. (2009). *Beliefs and illness: A model for healing.* Calgary, AB: 4th Floor Press.

Wright, L.M., & Leahey, M. (2013) 6th Ed. *Nurses and families: A guide to family assessment and intervention.* Philadelphia: FA Davis Co.

Wright, L.M., Watson, W.L., & Bell, J.M. (1996). *Beliefs: The heart of healing in families and illness.* New York: Basic Books.

CHAPTER 1

SUFFERING AND SPIRITUALITY IN EVERYDAY LIFE

Out of suffering have emerged the strongest souls; the most massive characters are seared with scars.
Kahlil Gibran

Spirituality does not come from religion. It comes from our soul.
Anthony Douglas Williams

It is in our ordinary, everyday life that our encounters with suffering and spirituality in the context of illness often become extraordinary experiences. So, what does constitute and characterize suffering? What are our spiritual beliefs and practices when illness arises? How does one define suffering and spirituality? How are they connected? How is spirituality different from religion, or is it?

To illustrate the complexities and the many possible and varied answers to these questions, I have included some brief stories of suffering and spirituality in the context of illness. Of course, these illness narratives offered by colleagues/friends and me are much more extensive and expansive than what the few pages in this chapter permit, but the poignancy of their thoughts are profound, even if short. Following their stories, I add my own story for consideration.

Personal Narratives of Suffering and Spirituality When Illness/Loss Arise

Deep suffering is what healthcare professionals typically encounter in their daily practice with patients/families. It becomes readily apparent through these brief narratives that deep suffering frequently occurs within the context of illness and/or loss in as many and varied experiences as there are lives. When deep suffering happens, it leaves a penetrating mark. And, for all in these stories, their lives have profoundly changed as they have attempted to give meaning and understanding to these experiences. Of course, there can be suffering with illness that is temporary, after which one returns to their usual lives, but this is not the case with deep suffering. Spiritual thoughts, ponderings, and changes in illness beliefs and behavior often followed closely behind their deep suffering and, in some instances, even accompanied the suffering.

In *Man's Search for Meaning*, Victor Frankl famously said, "tears bear witness that a man had great courage, the courage to suffer."

It is a curious reflection. As a young nursing

student, it was commonplace for us to record and read "the patient is in good spirits." Now it is rare, or non-existent, that an assessment of a patient's "spirit" would be recorded on patient charts. So, even when illness is present, it does not always mean that one's spirit is dampened. It may take time to be reclaimed as in this first illness narrative.

The first illness story is a poignant description of one couple's deep suffering, particularly the expectant mother, on the loss of their first pregnancy and baby. It is fitting that this narrative be the initial one in this chapter as this young woman also challenges our stereotypes about those who have an atheist world view, but still acknowledging their own spirituality, an important distinction.

"Earlier this year, my five-year-long struggle with infertility came to an end with the joyous news that my husband and I had finally conceived a child. We were stunned, elated, relieved, and scared, as most first-time parents are. After rounds of fertility treatments, months upon months of failure, and thousands of dollars spent, we had finally "succeeded."

We skipped into our Frist Trimester Screening full of hope and blissful ignorance. We left that small, clinical, non-descript room two hours and four ultrasounds later completely shattered. At fourteen-weeks, our baby—our first child, our dream for the future—had been diagnosed in utero with Trisomy-13. I'm sure the very pregnant nurse who gave us the diagnosis said a lot of things.

I'm sure she tried to comfort us as we stared, uncomprehending, at the written report I would come to know so well in the weeks that followed. But, I didn't hear any of it. My eyes kept landing on the protective hand she held over her own protruding belly, the vision of our fetus floating limply on the big screen TV behind the ultrasound technician clouding my mind.

Trisomy-13, we would learn, is the "rarest of the rare and worst of the worst" chromosomal abnormality a fetus can suffer. It occurs randomly in 1 in every 250,000 pregnancies without cause or warning. Our baby, with its severe deficiencies, would not survive outside the womb for more than a few pain-filled minutes. Our baby would not survive.

I had suffered in my life before that moment. Or, I thought I had. But, nothing in my experience could have prepared me for the all-consuming pain of carrying a child that would not live. As an atheist, I didn't have the comfort of platitudes. I wouldn't meet my baby in another life; I wouldn't visualize it happily frolicking in heaven, and I knew its inevitable death wasn't part of some larger plan. It wasn't a lesson for me to learn. It hadn't been sent to test my strength or faith.

Spirituality, to me, has always been internal. It's something within myself, not outside—it's the whole of who I am and how I connect to those around me. In suffering the loss of my child, those concepts solidified.

Motherhood is mainly a solitary endeavour. While I have the love and support of a caring and devoted husband, who I recognize also suffered this great loss, it was me who carried the child; who fed it and felt it flutter for the first time. And, in the end, on a cold table surrounded by machines waiting for the procedure to start, it was just me. Within myself, I had to say goodbye and feel the pain of the child's removal.

I changed in that moment, in a way I likely won't ever be able to fully describe. My soul changed forever and I know that the core of who I am will never be the same. Suffering the illness and death of my baby did that.

In the months that followed, I progressed slowly with the help of a good therapist, from being crippled by the loss, to accepting it, to being able to live alongside it. I healed, and continue to heal every day, as much as I can in every moment.

Outside support through the therapeutic process helped, but again it was down mostly to me. I had to make the therapy appointments, find the wherewithal to get dressed (I'll admit, I wore my pajamas on the first few visits), leave the house, and talk to a stranger about my greatest pain. She struggled at times with my atheism—something she initially wrongly assumed was a lack of spirituality. It left her searching for words of comfort that held no religious connotation. But, to her credit, she found them, and over time came to realize that my sense of spirit, my happy internal life, was exactly what had been wounded by my experience. I had lost the ability to be calm and comforted within my own mind, something I had always felt and treasured. That peaceful solitude, I was finally able to articulate, is my spirituality. My internal spirit.

Together, my therapist and I struggled through the PTSD, the noise of my cluttered and repetitious mind, a staggering number of tears, and all my fears of moving forward. As a witness to my suffering, she acknowledged the pain of my experience, the stress of dealing with the grief of my friends and family, and the casual cruelty of an insensitive world, and pushed me to first to reclaim my spirit—my internal calm—and then, finally, to entertain the possibility of moving on."

There is much to reflect upon and learn from this heart-rending narrative. This young woman recognized that this suffering was incomparable to previous suffering. Deep suffering, as she so profoundly states, was "soul changing." It reminds us that one aspect of healing is that our spirit or soul must heal in addition to having a peaceful mind, with peaceful thoughts. And, she offers a wonderful shout out to the healthcare professional who assisted her in reclaiming her spirit by eventually being able to acknowledge that one *can* identify as an atheist *and* experience spiritual distress. Fortunately, healing did and is taking place through "reclaiming" her spirit.

In this next narrative, another woman also dramatically describes and makes significant distinctions between what was previously thought of as suffering to the new experience of deep suffering. She discounts previous experiences she thought of as suffering, but were not as "soul searing and spirit killing" as this illness experience. Is this not another example of deep suffering, one that changes your life and relationships forever? And, understandably so! This horrific illness story brought a deepening of the spirit to an already 'deep soul.'

> *"Due to an increasingly malignant (adrenal) Cushings Syndrome, my immune debility and hormonal holocaust manifested in a series of illnesses over a two-year period: a ruptured spinal disc, diabetes, uncontrolled hypertension, disfiguring weight gain, muscular neuropathy, and osteoporosis. Following the adrenalectomy, I experienced surgically induced Addison's Disease (still do), a fractured fibula, and thyroid cancer. I continue to monitor bone masses that were "discovered" on one of these diagnostic forays.*
>
> *But, what, before my illnesses, I might have labeled "my suffering," I see in hindsight was only my anxiety, doubt, deep regret, disappointment, discouragement—not the soul searing, spirit killing that I now know as suffering. In another lexicon, suffering is a shape-shifter!"*

Suffering and Spirituality

I was incredibly moved by and stand in deep awe and respect for each of these powerful stories. One of the surprising experiences for me is that although I am familiar with these stories, to read them on paper gave them a new light, and a new understanding for me about deep suffering and spirituality. Both expressed to me that the writing of these illness narratives was cathartic and gave a clearer vision and meaning to their suffering and spirituality.

Now, I will add my own story of when I first experienced suffering and spirituality in everyday life. It was during my childhood when my English maternal grandmother, who lived with us, suffered chronic pain from rheumatoid arthritis. She had tremendous status and respect in our family by filling the role of "mother" by day while my mother worked outside the home with my father in our family business.

I observed the demoralizing deep suffering that one can experience from chronic pain, whether it be firsthand, as my grandmother suffered, or second-hand, as I emotionally suffered with her. I also learned that chronic pain controlled all our lives, especially how well my brother and I would behave on any given day, how much my grandmother was able to "mother," and how we children were invited to be more compassionate because of having a pain-sufferer in the family. My grandmother was the center of our family, but the chronic pain she suffered ruled even her. The disease severely disfigured her hands, caused her knees to be swollen much of the time, resulted in her walking with a limp, and dictated how well she was able to live her life on any given day. But, those disfigured hands made us apple pie, weeded our garden, and lifted numerous cups of tea while we exchanged stories of our lives and relationships with her. However, I do not recall as a child hearing *her* stories of suffering with chronic pain. Perhaps I did not listen. Perhaps these stories were not told. Perhaps I did not know what to ask as a child.

Now, even decades later, I have several questions that I would eagerly ask of my beloved grandmother if I could. What meaning did she give to this life of chronic pain? What did she believe was the best treatment or healing for her pain? What did she believe helped to soften her suffering? What made it worse? What made it better? What help or hindrance were her spiritual and religious beliefs? Did she pray about her pain? What did she believe we grandchildren did to help or hinder her pain? Which was worse: emotional, physical, or spiritual pain? And, what did she believe healthcare professionals did to help or hinder her pain? I wonder if conversations that may have included the answers to these questions would have contributed to some healing for both my grandmother and me.

THOUGHTS ABOUT THE ILLNESS NARRATIVES

From these very compelling and heartfelt stories, it seems clear that deep suffering is life-wrenching and life-altering, yet can even be life-giving. Suffering usually leads one on a spiritual journey or a turning toward their spiritual beliefs in their quest for meaning. In this quest, deep suffering and joy are inextricably connected and even surprisingly on the same side of the coin. "Even the most physical suffering is not strictly physical at all. It does not end in the physical realm where it began. It soaks into the heart and spreads. Suffering is finely connected to the versatile and permanent self, the spirit. Suffering is a spiritual matter." (Brickey, 2001, p. 47)

One recurring theme is that no one remains the same after deep suffering. Perhaps this is because suffering does not seem to come with an easy roadmap for finding our way to understanding its existence or why we suffer at all in life's journey. Even without a roadmap, perhaps one of the gifts of suffering is that it brings with it a particular depth and richness of thought. As one woman said: "I don't miss my illness, but I do miss the quality of thought. I was more removed from the world and its trivia." Yes, deep suffering does invite a particular depth of thought, a particular sobering and humbling opportunity for growth, for change, and for a possible openness or invitation to spirituality.

One person's deep suffering is not the same as another's, nor do we arrive at the same meaning that is derived from suffering experiences. Even within similar cultures and similar religious traditions, the meaning that each derives from their suffering can be vastly different. But, suffering does seem to have a constant companion with spirituality.

Definition of Deep Suffering

These poignant illness narratives and reflections of others plus my own, have compelled me to offer my definitions of deep suffering and spirituality for reference throughout the remainder of this text.

My current definition of deep suffering is: physical, emotional, or spiritual anguish, pain, or distress that changes one's life and relationships forever. Experiences of deep suffering can include: serious illness; loss; the forced exclusion from everyday life; the strain of trying to endure; acute or chronic pain; conflict, anguish, or interference with love in relationships when illness and/or loss arises.

Over the course of the last five years of my mother's life, she suffered and endured debilitating and limiting life experiences with Multiple Sclerosis. There were certain conversations we had that made a profound impact on me and have lingered over several years. One such conversation was on a day when I was wondering about the effect of my parents' move from their home in another city to the city where I currently live. The rationale for the move was that having our parents closer to us, my brother/sister-in-law and I could be of more help and assistance to them. However, I worried if my mother was missing her home and friends in this other city. So, one day I inquired, "Mom, do you miss Winnipeg?"

She responded with what became for me a great teaching moment. "No, Lorraine, I miss my life!"

Is it not the missing of a former life, or the missing of what one had hoped for in life, with or without a serious illness, that is part of deep suffering? Following periods of deep suffering, our lives as we knew them, *are* changed forever!

DEFINITION OF SPIRITUALITY

My current definition of spirituality is: whatever or whoever gives ultimate meaning and purpose in one's life that invites connection, intimacy, and particular ways of being in the world towards others and oneself. It is being aligned with one's own inner being, spirit, or one's soul, that is the seat of all inspiration, intuition, and wisdom.

I believe that everyone has a spirituality

or a particular way of being in the world. Others also embrace a religion. For the purposes of the discussion in this book, I have made a distinction between spirituality and religion, although for me in my everyday life, they fit well being integrated. It is apparent in the illness stories in this chapter that distinctions and integration of religion and spirituality are clearly exemplified. One did not have the need to identify their religion and one did not embrace any particular religion.

DEFINITION OF RELIGION

My current definition of religion is: the affiliation or membership in a particular faith community who share a set of beliefs, rituals, morals, and sometimes a health code centered on a defined Higher or Transcendent Power most frequently referred to as God.

Religion, at its best, provides a home for the nourishment and development of a spiritual life. Most often, this is the case, but sometimes it is not. Religious beliefs and practices can be a source of great comfort to those who suffer with serious illness and loss. However, it can also add to suffering if persons believe that their illness is due to not having lived a life in congruence with their religious beliefs or do not believe that their past deeds or behaviors are worthy of forgiveness or can be forgiven.

TAKEAWAYS FROM ILLNESS NARRATIVES

What are the takeaways from these powerful narratives? The first takeaway is the appreciation that deep suffering and spirituality are intricately connected. Another takeaway I believe is the need for ongoing development of our own spirituality that has the potential to assist us enormously when deep suffering arises, and particularly in later life when illness and loss tend to occur with greater frequency and regularity.

Another takeaway is that in our professional practice, we need to remember that "meaning-centered" conversations provide a critical boost and ability for individuals and families to cope and manage serious illness when their suffering is softened. It is even more important for those nearing the end of their lives. In my clinical practice with clients and their families, young and old, and even those persons with just a few weeks or months to live, they can benefit from finding meaning and value in their lives through therapeutic conversations with healthcare professionals who are able to soften their suffering. Talking *is* healing (Bell, 2016; Wright, 2015). It is never too late.

Thus, it is our great privilege as healthcare professionals to assist those suffering deeply with serious illness, loss, and grief to find meaning, purposefulness, intimacy, and connections in their new and altered 'everyday lives.' I offer this chapter and these stories as a way of hopefully inviting you, the reader, to a more personal reflection on your own suffering and spirituality. Your reflections will, I believe, open space to the Trinity Model presented in this text, and the examples of families with whom I have worked in my professional practice that are presented in the chapters that follow. By the conclusion of this book, particularly in Chapter 6, it will become apparent that in matters of suffering and spirituality, we cannot help but connect the personal and the professional.

REFERENCES

Bell, J.M. (2016). The central importance of therapeutic conversations in family nursing: Can talking be healing? *Journal of Family Nursing 22(4)*, 439–449 doi: 10.1177/1074840716680837

Brickey, W.E. (2001). *Making sense of suffering.* Salt Lake City: Deseret Book.

Wright, L. M. (2015). Brain science and illness beliefs: An unexpected explanation of the healing power of therapeutic conversations and the family interventions that matter. *Journal of Family Nursing, 21*, 186-205. doi:10.1177/1074840715575822

Chapter 2

Suffering and Illness

Suffering completely fills the human soul and conscious mind, no matter if the suffering is great or little.
Victor Frankl

Is suffering really necessary? Yes and no. If you had not suffered as you have, there would be no depth to you, no humility, no compassion.
Eckhart Tolle

"Why me?" Not Taking Suffering Personally and Accepting What Is

The first question many people ask when suffering with serious illness is "Why me?" Suffering seems to be the only human experience that evokes this question. Suffering seems to invite us to take it quite personally. If we won the lottery, would we ask, "Oh, why me? What did I do to deserve all this money?" On those happy, satisfying days, we don't seem to reflect on "Why me? What did I do to warrant being so happy?" In the instances of happiness and money, we tend to not ask questions, but instead make statements about how grateful and appreciative we are. Statements such as, "I'm so grateful for this windfall of money so that I can help my family" or "I just feel so happy with my life these days, all the hard work is paying off."

Questions of "why me" seem to flee when an abundance of happiness or excess money enters our lives, but we *do* tend to ask the "Why me" question when illness or loss befalls us. With experiences of illness suffering or loss, we focus on what have we done to bring this level of suffering into our lives.

Searching for the answer to "Why me?" can send some on a quest for the rest of their lives as they try to determine why their illness or loss did happen. We can blame our genetics, lifestyle, or even God for our suffering from illness or loss. But, the great enlightenment and wisdom comes when we realize that suffering really has nothing to do with "us," personally. It has to do with the larger human condition, our common humanity, and that to be alive is to know suffering. Suffering is not partial to any particular gender, race, or religion. It spares no one and favors no one. Suffering can visit the young as well as the old. We cannot go sideways in life to avoid suffering. No one escapes, except by challenging our constraining beliefs about suffering and asking different questions. Yes, suffering begs for explanation, but it is our *beliefs about illness suffering* that will either enhance or soften our suffering (Tolle, 2003; Wright & Bell, 2009).

To soften our suffering, we need to stop taking

suffering so personally, to change our questions and our thoughts.

What would happen to our experience of illness suffering if we were to ask, "Why *NOT* me?" In my clinical practice and personal life, I have met wise, learned, and insightful individuals who understand and believe that the universe is not selecting or choosing them to suffer, and consequently they tend to suffer less despite living with a serious illness. As one man suffering with life-threatening pancreatic cancer said to me "If I say 'why me,' does that mean I think others should have this awful illness and not me? No, that is not fair. I do not think we are 'chosen' to have a horrible illness. So, I say, 'why not me?" Would "Why *NOT* me?" paradoxically free us to allow healing to begin and our suffering to soften or even vanish? I believe so and have witnessed in my clinical practice that when an individual or family can ask the "Why not me?" question, healing has already begun.

Would a change in our question also invite a change in our beliefs about suffering? What would happen if we stopped resisting suffering and instead began accepting "what is" when illness or loss arises (Tolle, 2003; Wright, 2015)? What would happen if we acknowledged this experience as an essential and obligatory part of living, of being alive? For example, Eckhart Tolle (2005) suggests, "You can't argue with what is, with what you are experiencing. Well, you can, but if you do, you will suffer more."

(pg 184)

In other words, Tolle offers the useful notion that our suffering frequently arises from resisting "what is." When we resist, it usually has evolved from our constraining illness beliefs and the negative stories we have created out of those beliefs (Wright & Bell, 2009). Remember, it is never the particular illness or loss that generates our suffering, it is our constraining thoughts or beliefs about our current situation. The illness or loss is "what is," the facts, the truth, but the suffering arises when we defend, argue, become angry, or disagree with what has occurred in our life. These are all various forms of "resistance." Of course, there are times when our life does not go the way we had hoped, wanted, or desired. Understandably, we can experience serious illness, loss, and/disability with sadness, despair, or grief. But, these emotions are different from resistance! Resistance can trigger the amygdala into a stress response of negative and discouraging beliefs about an illness experience because the amygdala is prepared to activate in response to fearful or potentially threatening inputs (Wright, 2015). By challenging constraining illness beliefs, we quiet the amygdala in the brain. When the amygdala is quieted, suffering is softened.

This idea of not resisting "what is" has expanded my understanding of suffering in the context of illness. For example, in my practice, family members often make comments such as "I haven't been a bad person, therefore it's not fair that I have this illness" or "If only I hadn't been so stressed with my work, this heart attack would not have happened." These kinds of comments are based on illness beliefs that are focused on the past, which invariably invites suffering.

Alternatively, patients and families often make comments about the future: "how will we be able to care for Mother at home?" or "how is he going to be able to work now with this disability?" or "How will I go on with my life if my child dies?" Questions about the future also tend to invite suffering. If one can primarily live being more focused on the present moment, even with an experience of serious illness, accepting "what is," rather than focusing on the past or future, and challenging any constraining beliefs, there is no suffering. Therefore, in my clinical practice, rather than focusing on the past or future about illness or loss, I try instead to bring forth the illness narrative; acknowledge and witness suffering; gently challenge constraining illness beliefs; and then observe the healing outcome that often occurs from softening or diminishing suffering.

A distinction needs to be made, however, that "accepting what is" does not imply accepting one's specific illness or loss, but rather that we accept the condition in which we find ourselves on any particular day. When one enters into this kind of acceptance, it allows them to feel whatever it is they are feeling at that moment. For example, if today you are experiencing difficulty walking post-surgery from an illness, it is the acceptance of today's "immobility" that you shouldn't resist. Or, if you have recently experienced the death of a loved one and on this day you are feeling immensely sad, you don't resist this emotion, but rather acknowledge the emotion of deep sadness as part of your grieving. Whatever you accept completely will take you to a place of peace, even sometimes including the acceptance that you cannot accept, that sometimes you are in resistance.

If action needs to be taken with a particular issue with regard to managing an illness or loss, the idea or inspiration for solutions will come from a peaceful state, rather than one of suffering and angst. This concept may sound idealistic, but I have witnessed this transformation from suffering to surrender in my clinical practice and the peace that follows. By peace is meant there is great focus on the present moment, rather than letting the mind live in the past or future, which can directly or indirectly invite more suffering. Resistance is such a large part of the experience of suffering in relation to one's constraining illness beliefs, that is… resisting "what is." Resistance stifles inspiration! This new understanding has been a helpful addition to my clinical practice and is benefiting the individuals and families I have the privilege of assisting. It has also benefitted me in my personal life.

Finally, these ideas of "not taking suffering personally" and "accepting what is" were not ideas that I wrote about in the first edition of *Spirituality, Suffering, and Illness: Ideas for Healing* in 2005. This is evidence that I continue to learn and evolve in my ideas about suffering through the insights of spiritual teachers, such as Eckhart Tolle; my own experiences of anguish and suffering; and the heartfelt experiences of suffering I have encountered with many more patients/families since the writing of the previous edition. Suffering is part of living, so I continue to learn from it, try to not take it so personally, and accept what is.

DEFINITION OF DEEP SUFFERING

The physical, emotional, or spiritual anguish, pain, or distress that changes one's life and relationships forever. Experiences of deep suffering can include: serious illness; loss; the forced exclusion from everyday life; the strain of trying to endure; acute or chronic pain; conflict, anguish, or interference with love in relationships when illness and/or loss arise.

SOFTENING SUFFERING IS THE HEART OF CLINICAL PRACTICE

As healthcare professionals, how should

suffering be addressed in our clinical practice? I submit that softening suffering, particularly deep suffering, is the center, the essence, and the heart of healthcare professionals' clinical practice. Therefore, the ethical and obligatory goal of every healthcare professional must be to soften or diminish (and hopefully heal) emotional, physical, and/or spiritual suffering of patients and their family members. I believe that the softening of suffering has always been the heart of clinical practice, though it's not recognized as such. Reed (2003), perplexed by the lack of attention to suffering by healthcare professionals, offers this poignant comment:

"How strange it seems that suffering and its relief, which are central to the mission of healthcare, are mentioned so infrequently in many hospitals and within the health-care delivery system.

"Although there is much talk in clinical conferences about treatment strategies, physical symptom management, and patient care outcomes, it would be quite remarkable to discover a case conference planned to address "The Suffering of John T, Room 310." The successes of modern science convey the impression that suffering has been conquered, but sensitive observation in any health-care environment demonstrates that suffering is pervasively present." (p. 4).

Conversations about suffering are not routinely brought forth in healthcare professionals' encounters with families experiencing serious illness, except perhaps in areas of palliative care and oncology that have been leading the way (Ferrell & Coyne, 2008). What prevents or impedes healthcare professionals to engage their patients in conversations about suffering? In this chapter, I offer my own reflections of this relational phenomena; examine what exists in the professional literature; and give professional and personal examples that provide clues to answer this question, specifically the insights from a research study my colleagues and I conducted, which examined actual therapeutic conversations about illness suffering.

Suffering is raw, personal, and deep. Suffering is not partial to any particular gender, race, or religion. Suffering spares no one, and favors no one. Suffering greets the young as well as the old. And, suffering has a very demanding dimension. It continually begs for explanation about why suffering has occurred and how it can be endured. Suffering can mean to experience, undergo, or tolerate anguish, grief, loss, and/or unwanted or unanticipated change. This type of suffering within the context of illness needs to be told and talked about. However, too often patients and family members are encouraged to only tell their medical story or narrative. The medical narrative means to discuss the disease or condition, complete with medication, dosages, and tests, while the illness narrative is the story of suffering and the effects of this suffering on the individual, their relationships, and their world.

The capacity of healthcare professionals to witness the stories of suffering in families is central to providing care; it is frequently the genesis of hope and healing, but it is not easy to listen to heartfelt and heart wrenching illness suffering. In working with individuals and families, helping professionals have an important opportunity to invite and witness stories, within which a "domain of spirituality" is encountered. This journey into spirituality manifests itself in the "offering of reverencing, compassion, and love between and among family members and therapists." (Wright, 1999, p. 75) In the inviting and witnessing of stories, the spirituality that is embedded in our lived experience of the world addresses both clinicians and patients/families.

THE EMERGENCE OF SUFFERING IN ILLNESS

Serious illness invites a wake-up call about life. Serious illness comes in many forms such as chronic, life threatening, or mental illness. It arouses the need to be known, to be heard, and to be validated—the need to know that one's life matters in the life of someone else and that the life one is living and has lived is and has been worthwhile (Frank, 1994). These needs fuel the telling of individual and family members' experiences with illness. And, these illness experiences have become known as illness stories or narratives (Kleinman, 1988).

It is within these illness stories that suffering looms. Most healthcare professionals are always in the midst of a person's encounter with illness. They have the privileged opportunity to bring forth illness narratives in their therapeutic conversations with persons suffering with serious illness. But, it is deep suffering that is most frequently encountered by healthcare professionals where one's life and relationships are changed forever by experiences of serious illness, loss, and/or disability. Chesla (2005) prefers to describe this change in everyday life when a chronic illness appears as a "breakdown." This breakdown, she suggests, contributes to individuals/families suffering deeply over their losses. There's no question that the changes in everyday life brought forth by serious illness trigger deep suffering and have the ability to create particular kinds of illness stories.

But, Eckhart Tolle cautions us as healthcare professionals to distinguish the illness narrative or "the story" from "the facts." Too often, our patients/families create an unhelpful or even a suffering story from the facts. The facts are normally the particular illness or condition with which they have been diagnosed. But, then, stories unfold around these conditions that are often unhelpful, negative, and victim-based, arising from their illness beliefs. In the context of illness, these stories invite further suffering, rather than dealing with the facts and responding accordingly. This is similar to the idea that I recently wrote in a paper about brain science and illness beliefs, specifically that the brain has a negativity bias (Wright, 2015).

The following illness narrative is a poignant and sad account of a young thirty-four-year-old woman's experience of suffering with psychosis. Her understanding of Eckhart Tolle's (2005) powerful notion that we do not have to believe all our thoughts, or at least not take them seriously, can be very empowering and paved the path for her illness healing. This young woman was able to take her understanding of her psychotic experiences even further by recognizing that it was when she could be devoid of negative, blaming stories or thoughts that she encountered her own spiritual awakening and the softening of her suffering. No doubt, this young woman also brought forth courage and resilience from deep inside, or what we might call her 'spirit,' to overcome such traumatic childhood experiences that were transformed into a full-blown psychotic episode. But, eventually, she was able to soften her suffering and found peace of mind through observing her thoughts and refraining from believing all of her thoughts and the negative stories that emerged from them. Although she experienced traditional medical treatment for psychosis with hospitalization and psychotropic medications, it is fascinating that she attributes her greatest growth and overcoming her psychosis to her ability and capacity to suspend her negative, blaming, suffering stories. This enabled her suffering to soften and invited her "spiritual awakening," as she describes it.

> *"I grew up with limited exposure to any form of spirituality or religion. Instead, it turned out that suffering was my spiritual teacher. It took me many years to process the episode of psychosis I experienced as a teenager. I now see it as not just as mental illness, but part of a spiritual process.*
>
> *The build-up of suffering started in childhood. When I was very young, around five years old, I witnessed violence between my parents. While disturbing for anyone, from a child's perspective it is also traumatic.*
>
> *The memory of this came back to me only as an adult. My emotions remained buried though and I carried a lot of sadness and confusion. I would switch between subdued and attention-seeking behaviour. Without the vocabulary to express or make sense of these disturbing emotions, there was a continuous feeling that something was wrong. I felt I had to put on a mask to fit in and get by. Anything else would force me to face the pain.*
>
> *Over time, the emotions that were left undealt with grew stronger. An unhappy child turned into a suicidal teenager. By seventeen, the cumulative pressure of suffering was more than could be contained. The limit of*

suppression had finally been hit and I was ready to erupt.

Almost overnight, I was drawn into delusions of different realities. I was overtaken by a desperate need to escape. Petrified by the people around me. Not knowing what they wanted from me. Having no awareness that it was my erratic and unusual behaviour that had changed, and friends and family were simply reacting to it. Painful memories of the past came up as real as if they were happening all over again. Terror, fear, frustration, confusion all re-visited. My spiritual teacher was strong and fierce.

The world looked very different through the eyes of psychosis. Everything was a symbol. Colours signified safety or danger. Everything everyone did or said held some kind of hidden meaning—what was it trying to tell ME? I became completely centred around myself. So much so, I believed the whole world had been created for me. It was such a strong thought that it felt like a sudden realization. Every person I'd ever seen or known was an actor put there to teach me something. I believed that my "real family" would eventually come to take me back home. It brought such relief. Suddenly, everything was ok. This rationale explained why nothing had ever felt quite right. In an instant, the past became insignificant.

It was in this moment of perceived limbo between two realities that I let go of all thought... that is, all thoughts that had invited deep suffering. Or, perhaps, thought let go of me. I was without burden or worry of any kind, when I felt a sensation of aliveness from the inside my body. As my mind became free of negative thoughts, my whole body was literally vibrating with joy—I could feel a tangible sensation of peace, what I later recognized as "The peace that passeth all understanding."

I later learnt that it was my thoughts or beliefs that created deep suffering that evolved to particular negative stories I would tell myself. I had been continually interpreting the world through the eyes of my child self—as unsafe and hostile, and therefore I experienced it as so. While thought is indispensable for practical purposes, so much of it takes us away from true contentment, awakening, enlightenment, or knowing God. There was a significant enough gap between an old story and a new story, where I felt truly at peace. All the suffering from childhood, accumulating to psychosis, was so unbearably painful, it pushed me to an extreme and I had no choice but to let go of it.

Many years later, when I encountered Eckhart Tolle's books on spirituality, it made sense to me that through quieting the mind, we can feel an inner body aliveness and experience spiritual awakening. My suffering was a harsh teacher of this and forced me into this state, but it also led me to a gentler teaching in the form of Tolle, by which I can invite the stillness in and have moments of entering that state voluntarily.

My deep suffering led to illness, which

offered further intense suffering. My unhappy story had become so unbearable that I finally rested in a space completely free of any negative thoughts. Instead, I experienced the deepest part of who I really am, beyond the person, I experienced my soul. Not all stories are so unhappy or lead to such an extreme consequence. This was my curse and my blessing—the grace of a spiritual awakening. Fortunately, I have been psychosis free for a few years now. But, I have to be ever vigilant for the re-emergence of negative stories that can invite me back into deep suffering. My life as an author seems to be the perfect outlet for me to keep my own suffering stories at bay while I create other stories."

This illness narrative is touching, moving, and inspiring as this young woman's deep suffering began to dissolve when she directly experienced Tolle's insight that for some persons "suffering is necessary until you realize it is no longer necessary."

Knowing that deep suffering can be uncovered through the bringing forth of illness stories enables us to assist patients/families in their illness journey by engaging in more hopeful and healing illness stories. In other words, we need to stick to the facts and help family members (and ourselves) resist creating unhelpful, negative stories filled with constraining beliefs about the cause and/or impact of a particular illness but rather generate stories of hopefulness and healing. Illness stories of hope and healing are filled with facilitating illness beliefs, plus the strengths, and resources that families have perhaps forgotten or suppressed. Bringing these overlooked and neglected individual/family strengths and resources is perhaps one of our most empowering clinical practices. At the end of a meeting with a couple seeking ideas about how to live with chronic pain, the wife said to me: "I always know that I will feel better when we meet with you because you remind us that we do have strengths that we have forgotten as chronic pain takes all of our attention."

But, paradoxically, for hope and healing to occur, illness stories must first be brought forth, as well as any constraining illness beliefs embedded in those stories. We must ask therapeutic questions to understand each family member's beliefs about the effect, impact, and changes in a person's life and relationships. Questions such as "What changes, if any, have there been in your life since you were diagnosed with your serious illness?" "What has been the effect of this illness upon your marriage, your family?" These types of questions address the deep suffering that is being endured and the systemic effects of that suffering. Sometimes, questions can be even more specific about deep suffering by simply asking: "Who in the family is suffering the most?"

RELATIONAL EFFECT OF ILLNESS SUFFERING

It has been surprising and enlightening to me that most frequently the person who is suffering the most is *not* the person with the illness diagnosis. The responses to these types of questions quickly confirm that deep suffering *is* the illness experience. But, unfortunately, it is not typically part of most healthcare professionals' therapeutic conversations with patients/families to ask these types of questions.

This notion that it is often another family member who is suffering the most was dramatically brought home to me during the privilege I had of meeting and interviewing a lovely Brazilian family while lecturing at the University of Sao Paulo and the Federal University of Sao Paulo.

Ever since the renowned film *Titanic*, Leonardo DiCaprio captured me with his superb acting, charm, and good looks. Yes, he has been my favorite and he has been only Leonardo ever since. But, when I met this Brazilian family, another Leonardo came into my life and replaced Leonardo, the actor.

The family consisted of the mother, age 53, who was diagnosed with lymphosarcoma; father, age 47, and their two children, Fabiana, age 24, and Leonardo, age 20. The mother sat in a wheelchair during the interview, appearing very thin and wearing a scarf to cover her head that was left bald as a result of chemotherapy treatments. The mother and father had been married for twenty years, but now separated for five years. Surprisingly, although they were separated, they were still very "married" as evidenced by their descriptions of their relationship as being "closer," with more "friendship" and "caring."

After our initial greetings to one another, I asked the family a variety of assessment and interventive questions (Wright & Leahey, 2013) to invite their illness narrative and ascertain how they were experiencing this hard journey with a serious, life-threatening illness. For example, I explored the roles in the family by asking who was caring for their mother at home. To my amazement, Fabiana answered that it was Leonardo, her brother. I told Leonardo that in Canada, I had never met a young twenty-year-old son who cared for his ill mother.

Leonardo's name was offered again when I asked the question, *"Who in the family is suffering the most?"* The son affirmed other family members' perspective that he definitely was the one with the most anguish in this experience of his mother's illness. Fabiana offered the explanation that Leonardo was suffering the most because he was the "keychain" to his mother. Leonardo and his father agreed with this perception. Their responses validated once again my own observations with numerous families that the family member suffering the most is frequently *not* the one with the illness diagnosis.

Through further therapeutic questions, Leonardo revealed that he accepted his role willingly to care for his mother. And, in the caring for his mother, he had even discovered a new interest in "gastronomy" (cooking) that he wished to pursue when his mother was well enough for him to obtain further training. The family was optimistic about the mother's prognosis because of her positive response to chemotherapy treatments.

At the end of our meeting, I offered the family a few commendations (Houger, Limacher & Wright, 2006). Specifically, I offered them the idea that I believed that the caring and devotion they showed to their mother and wife had also contributed to her healing, in addition to the chemotherapy treatments. They all agreed.

I gave special attention to Leonardo by telling him that I would always remember him and that he was much more handsome and was doing something much more worthwhile than Leonardo the actor. He smiled profusely, as did all family members. Yes, *this* Leonardo is *my new favorite one* because he willingly gave so much of his young life and love to his mother during this very trying time. It was indeed an honor to have met Leonardo and his family.

I am also very grateful to my colleague/friend, Dr. Margareth Angelo of the University of Sao Paulo, who patiently and caringly provided translation between the family and me for that interview.

SUFFERING AND FAMILIES

The description above of the lovely family I interviewed in Brazil illustrates once again that illness is a family affair and all family members suffer, some more, some less. Therefore, it compels us as healthcare professionals to attend to the entire family with regards to suffering, and not just the person diagnosed with a particular illness.

If healthcare professionals would embrace just this one belief, that illness is a family affair, it would change the face of clinical practice with families and minimize suffering (Wright & Leahey, 1999; Wright & Leahey, 2013). No one person in a family experiences cancer, epilepsy, or heart disease. All family members are influenced by the illness and reciprocally, all family members can contribute to the healing of an illness.

On a personal note, if healthcare professionals had embraced the notion that illness is a family affair and consequently all family members suffer, it would have provided much needed healing for my family and me. During my mother's five-year ordeal with Multiple Sclerosis (MS), she received competent caring by nurses, physicians, and other healthcare professionals for her physical suffering. But, my mother's emotional and spiritual suffering was rarely addressed. Nor was the suffering of my father, other family members, and my own. During the last year of my mother's life, she had become a quadriplegic and experienced frequent severe pain in her hands. After one telephone call from my father, I was so struck by his words. "We were having a great day until the pain returned—now nothing seems to be helping. I've given your mother all the pain medication and more that I can. I'm rubbing her hands with that new ointment. It's very tough to watch her suffer. I've lost my appetite and won't be having supper tonight." Is illness not a family affair? Who was suffering the most emotionally, my mother or my father? And, who the most physically?

But, families frequently discover their own unique self-care solutions to softening their suffering. We need to take the opportunity to explore their self-soothing options to soften suffering. For example, we can ask the question, "What have you found that helps to soften your suffering during your treatments?" One dear friend who was in the mist of chemotherapy treatments for breast cancer told me, "There must be fifty ways to suck your thumb! Some of my favorites are: stay in bed, have a very hot bubble bath, read 500 pages of a good book, watch TV (nothing more violent than *Murder, She Wrote*). Oh, and another way I suck my thumb is comfort food." Yes, there are many ways to "suck your thumb" or soften suffering. As we collaborate with patients/families, we can learn from each other about what works and what doesn't!

SUFFERING, SPIRITUALITY, AND THEOLOGY

Suffering invites us into the spiritual domain. A shift to an emphasis on spirituality is frequently the most profound response to suffering from serious illness. If healthcare professionals are to be helpful, we must acknowledge that suffering and, often, the senselessness of it are ultimately spiritual issues. A more in-depth discussion of spirituality and illness will be presented in Chapter 3.

The experience of suffering often becomes transposed to one of spirituality as individuals/family members try to make meaning out of their suffering and distress. Suffering leads one into the spiritual domain as the big questions of life are faced (Wright, 1999; Wright & Bell, 2009). Questions such as "Why has this illness happened to me?" "Why do some people die before their time?" or "What am I supposed to learn from this suffering?"

Many beliefs and ideas exist about the purpose, lessons, and reasons for suffering. The medical perspective claims that suffering occurs in response to pain and illness; occurs as a response to the meaning of symptoms and occurs when the impending destruction of the person is perceived and to remove the threat is to remove the suffering (Morse, 2000).

Addressing the issue of what lessons can be learned from suffering, Anne Morrow Lindbergh

(1973) wrote one of her most oft quoted statements: "I do not believe that sheer suffering teaches. If suffering alone taught, all the world would be wise since everyone suffers. To suffering must be added mourning, understanding, patience, love, openness and the willingness to remain vulnerable." (pg 3)

Theological perspectives suggest that suffering has redemptive and transformative qualities. For example, Whitney (1966) attempts to put a kindlier face to suffering by suggesting certain benefits. "No pain that we suffer, no trial that we experience is wasted. It ministers to our education, to the development of such qualities as patience, faith, fortitude and humility. All that we suffer and all that we endure, especially when we endure it patiently, builds up our characters, purifies our hearts, expands our souls, and makes us more tender and charitable." (p.211)

Suffering does change us, and often for the better. Frequently, we have a deepened compassion, a more tender heart, or become less judgmental. But, suffering can also invite bitterness over losses, confusion about life's abrupt changes, anger over what might have been, and even competitiveness over what type of suffering is the most severe. These varying responses to suffering are all based on the stories we have created from our particular illness beliefs.

SUFFERING AND LANGUAGE IN HEALTHCARE

Unfortunately, attention to suffering has not increased in our current healthcare systems. This may be related to the perspective many healthcare professionals assert that their purpose is to cure patients with the application of scientific knowledge, techniques, and skills. It could also be related to shifting societal beliefs, particularly in North America, that values the pursuit of happiness and avoidance of suffering. These changing societal beliefs have also resulted in a change in our language when talking with patients and families. Instead of inquiring about illness suffering, healthcare professionals tend to use more upbeat and positive language with questions such as "How are you coping with your illness?" or "How are you adjusting?" The writer Barbara Ehrenreich criticized the cultural trend of positive thinking in her book *Smile or Die* (2009), where she condemned the 'bright-siding' of breast cancer in the developed world. It's difficult to escape the triumphalist talk of illness as a journey, she says, destined to end in the revitalisation of one's life, career, relationships and character. This kind of illness narrative excludes those who don't witness much personal growth, or those who don't recover fully or at all and do not enter into the "survivor club" of cancer victims. It is those who cannot return to their former selves and/or do not recover from their illness that often experience the most intense suffering as they struggle to find new meaning and new acceptance of themselves and by their loved ones of their altered life.

As one young man said to me during our therapeutic conversations together when we discussed his suffering from chronic pain, "At last someone is calling it what it is. I *do* suffer; it saps my spirit and I'm tired of hearing how well I'm coping." Here is a profound example where this young man teaches us that before illness healing can begin, acknowledging and witnessing suffering needs to occur. And, he connected suffering and spirituality.

The experience or depth of one person's suffering is never the same as someone else's. Suffering experiences cannot be compared, but unfortunately comparisons are made about which sufferings we believe are the most horrific. Is breast cancer of a young thirty-three-year-old mother more devastating than a brain tumor of a ten-year-old boy? As Nouwen (1992) so eloquently offers, "I am deeply convinced that each human being suffers in a way no other human being suffers... in the final analysis, your pain and my pain are so deeply personal that comparing them can bring scarcely any consolation or comfort." Recognizing that each person's suffering is unique and that attempting to have persons "count their blessings" can inadvertently trivialize suffering from illness.

Through highly privileged therapeutic conversations between health professionals and family members, it is readily acknowledged that suffering, illness beliefs, and spirituality are close cousins (Wright, 1999). They are so intertwined that it becomes difficult, or near impossible, to discuss or attend to one without attending to the others. (I have extended these ideas even further and offered the Trinity Model in Chapter 4).

SUFFERING AND ILLNESS RESEARCH

Frank (1994) suggests the primary lesson the ill have to offer is the "pedagogy of suffering." These teachings compel us to offer healing spiritual care practices that relieve deep suffering. But, what spiritual care practices are most beneficial to those who suffer? This compels healthcare professionals, or so it should, to conduct research to further our knowledge about which spiritual care practices actually do diminish or soften suffering.

To conduct research about illness suffering, I believe it is essential that we first acknowledge the dramatic difference in daily living between healthcare professionals and those in their care. The seriously ill and their family members live in a world that is profoundly dissident from healthcare professionals. The ill and their family members experience a world where deep suffering often becomes a constant companion, and frequently a tormenting and agonizing companion. This suffering manifests itself in many ways. For example, strained family relationships, forced exclusion from everyday life, and the loss of one's former life become commonplace.

The alleviation of deep suffering has always been the cornerstone of caring. All forms of caring aim, in one way or another, to soften suffering. But, what is the best way to care for those who are suffering? What do the seriously ill and their family members convey about their suffering in conversations with healthcare professionals? Listen to the suffering of a woman in her late forties experiencing the serious illness of Amyotrophic Lateral Sclerosis (ALS).

"I have suffered so many losses. In the eight months since my diagnosis, my legs, left hand and arm are paralyzed and my right hand is deteriorating. My capability of speech is gone and I am having trouble swallowing. I depend on everyone to do almost everything for me. But, this is just the summary of the physical list. What I have really lost is _me_! It is like everything I love is being moved out of my reach. Yet, I am still here in the presence of my life, unable to participate."

Suffering does not occur in a vacuum or in isolation. Suffering is linked to and intertwined with the beliefs that one holds about their illness. A belief is the "truth" of a subjective reality that influences biopsychosocial-spiritual structure and functioning (Wright & Bell, 2009). Individual illness beliefs of patients and family members are involved in both the experience of suffering and in making inferences of suffering. Certain beliefs may conserve or maintain an illness; others may exacerbate symptoms; others may soften suffering (Wright & Bell, 2009). For example, what family members and healthcare professionals believe about their prognosis, diagnosis, or treatment and healing can enhance or soften suffering. For a more in-depth understanding of the power of illness beliefs on enhancing or softening suffering, I refer you to my co-authored book *"Beliefs and Illness: A Model for Healing* (Wright & Bell, 2009).

From my own clinical practice with individuals/families and research conducted by myself or my healthcare professional colleagues, I have come to strongly believe that talking about illness experiences can often soften or diminish emotional, physical, and spiritual suffering (Bell, 2016; Sveinbjarnardottir, Svavarsdottir, & Wright, 2013; Wacharasin, 2010; Wright & Bell, 2009). To me, talking and listening to illness stories in purposeful therapeutic conversations becomes the context from which suffering can be softened and healing begins. Therefore, I believe that the best way to understand suffering is to examine actual conversations of illness sufferers and their healthcare professionals. I believe that cellular and "soulular" changes occur through these conversations. Our network of conversations and our relationships can contribute to the enhancement or softening of deep suffering from illness experiences.

Therefore, it is imperative that we connect the importance of intervention illness research with suffering. However, researchers immediately encounter significant challenges when embarking on research about suffering. How can the profound, human experience of suffering, particularly the suffering that accompanies serious illness, be fully appreciated and understood when examining interventions? What nursing behaviors can potentially enhance suffering? Perhaps the two most difficult questions for family nurse researchers are: "Can the profound experience of suffering be researched? (Frank, 2001). And conversely, can research contribute to further suffering?" Many researchers also strive to see if one can measure suffering. Moules (2010) reminds us that the phenomena of suffering, particularly grief, can never be measured or, in some ways, ever articulated. Suffering is a profound human experience that invariably escapes our ability to quantify it.

To date, most research has revealed descriptions of the experience of suffering and what has *not* been done to soften suffering. Frank (2001) argues that some aspects of suffering remain unspeakable. However, I believe the portions of suffering that can be spoken may be lessened when there is acknowledgment, witnessing, or "just listening" (Frank, 1998) of the ill person.

Suffering can be researched without contributing further to an individual's suffering if we fully engage with our patients and family members who are living with suffering. Chesla (2005) offers the possibility that the more we engage and pay attention to the everyday lives of families who are experiencing chronic illness and remain open to their suffering *and* their possibilities, the better we become as researchers, clinicians, and human beings. I concur.

In lectures and workshops that I offer worldwide, the poignant question is often asked, "How does a researcher or clinician listen to such suffering and remain detached?" My answer is always, "Why would we as researchers, or clinicians, or educators want to remain detached from another's suffering?" I am familiar with the arguments that researchers offer about the need to remain detached and distant from the topic and subjects being researched. Could our research not take on a more human and humane dimension if we allowed ourselves to be touched and moved by suffering? If a better understanding of which aspects of therapeutic conversations can potentially heal suffering, then the importance of routinely inviting these conversations of suffering and involving family members in healthcare can be further advocated and admonished.

INTERVENTION RESEARCH TO SOFTEN SUFFERING

Conducting research that examines the actual therapeutic conversations between families and healthcare professionals can point the way to learning, identifying, and confirming those clinical practices that indeed soften suffering and promote hope and healing. In so doing, we will move beyond research that only defines and describes suffering.

One context for conducting research that examined actual therapeutic conversations was within our Family Nursing Unit (FNU), a unique outpatient clinic, situated within the Faculty of Nursing, University of Calgary, which focused on clinical scholarship and advanced nursing practice with families suffering with serious illness (Bell, 2008; Gottlieb, 2007). I had the privilege of being the Director of this clinic for some twenty years (1982 – 2002) before its closure in 2007, after twenty-five years of operation. Families who were seen at the FNU were experiencing difficulties with serious illness. Faculty and graduate students collaborated and consulted with families to alleviate emotional, physical, relational, and/or spiritual suffering. Direct involvement with the nursing care of families enabled a focus of inquiry on examining the practice, offering descriptions of the practice, and continuously learning from families resulting in the discovery, organization, analysis, synthesis, and transmission of knowledge about caring practices with families experiencing illness. The relationship between practice scholarship and research became a circular interactional phenomenon where new understanding changed practice and changed practice invited new research questions. One of the results of our various research projects resulted in two advanced practice models, namely the Illness Beliefs Model (Wright & Bell, 2009) and the Trinity Model that I fully discuss in Chapter 4.

One of the first family intervention projects conducted in the FNU involved recruiting families who were experiencing hypertension (Duhamel, 1994). This study focused on therapeutic conversations with families experiencing hypertension. A multiple case study was designed and found that families who received family level interventions reported a decrease in symptoms in the hypertensive family member and improved family relationships (Duhamel, 1994; Duhamel, Watson, & Wright, 1994), leading the researcher to hypothesize about the usefulness of family systems interventions as a method of stress reduction.

Robinson's (1994) oft quoted and referenced qualitative grounded theory study examined the process and outcomes of interventions with families experiencing chronic illness. Her study revealed two major components of therapeutic change from the families' perspective are: creating the circumstances for change and moving beyond/overcoming problems (Robinson & Wright, 1995). Specifically, the nurses' act of bringing the family together and creating a sense of comfort and trust were the fundamental behaviors that enabled family members to convey their illness experiences. By providing a context for sharing among family members of their illness experiences, intense emotions are legitimized. Expressing the impact of the illness on the family and, reciprocally, the influence of the family on the illness, gives validation and voice to their experiences and thereby are healing practices that reduce suffering. Robinson (1998) also uncovered that even though illness affects all family members, it does not affect all family members equally. It was the women in this study who were suffering the most regardless if they were the one with the diagnosis, or their spouse or child. The publication of these research findings by Robinson and myself (Robinson & Wright, 1995) in the *Journal of Family Nursing* continues to rank as one of the most frequently cited publications in the twenty-plus-year history of the journal. This indicates to me that healthcare professionals, particularly nurses in this case, are eager to learn what particular therapeutic practices make a difference to families who are suffering and this study points the way.

Tapp's (1997; 2001, 2004) qualitative hermeneutic study explored the therapeutic conversations between nurses and families experiencing ischemic heart disease within the FNU. These therapeutic conversations moved beyond social conversations and were purposeful, deliberate, and healing. She uncovered that the conversations between nurses and families were about healthy lifestyles; family support; uncertainty and death. When spaces were created for these therapeutic conversations, conditions emerged for healing to occur. By engaging in these particular types of conversations with families experiencing heart disease, suffering was softened when possibilities for making sense of the illness and suffering were revealed.

A qualitative hermeneutic study by Moules (2000; 2002; 2009) explored the use of therapeutic letters within the clinical practice at the FNU. Her thoughtful and illuminating findings suggest that therapeutic letters written by nurses and mailed to families following family meetings have the potential for further healing and minimizing suffering. One of the most helpful guidelines for writing therapeutic letters emerged from Moules' findings was to recognize the "cries of the wounded" in the letters to acknowledge that the family's suffering has been heard.

Hougher Limacher (2003) further contributed to our knowledge by conducting a hermeneutic research study to better understand the family systems nursing intervention of 'commendations' (Wright & Bell, 2009). Commending patients and family members on their strengths, resources, and competencies in the midst of illness, asking reflective questions, and expanding the therapeutic relationship all serve to create a context for healing. But, it was Limacher's suggestion that it is the 'goodness' embedded in commendations that I, too, believe invites healing.

McLeod's (2003) hermeneutic inquiry was undertaken to explore the meaning of spirituality and spiritual care practices as practiced in the FNU. She concluded from this study that spiritual care practices must include conversations about the meaning of illness in families' lives and relationships, conversations about suffering, plus mentoring and life experiences (McLeod & Wright, 2008). This study emphasized that suffering embodies an obligation to respond to the spiritual; and to recognize that practices to create space for spiritual conversations include creating a sanctuary for stories of suffering to be heard and the use of rituals in acknowledging the sacred.

Another hermeneutic phenomenology research study by West (2011) examined illness suffering in families experiencing childhood cancer. Family process research methods were also used to analyze videotaped therapeutic conversations conducted in the FNU and included post-intervention family and clinician interviews. Findings suggest that the illness suffering of families is characterized in part by loss of family normalcy and particular family interventions were reported to lessen illness suffering. Those included: offering new interpretations of suffering; commending family strengths; acknowledging illness suffering; and eliciting the experiences of family members in the presence of other family members (West, Bell, Woodgate, & Moules, 2015).

RESEARCH SPECIFICALLY ADDRESSING ILLNESS SUFFERING IN THERAPEUTIC CONVERSATIONS

One study in our outpatient FNU focused entirely on conversations of illness suffering between nurses and families. The goal of this particular research project was to examine the nature of illness conversations that bring forth experiences of suffering and/or healing. It was externally funded by the Social Sciences and Humanities Research Council of Canada with members of the research team being Lorraine Wright, Janice Bell, and Nancy Moules, and two graduate students. This research project was a hermeneutic, interpretive study (Moules et al, 2015; Moules et al, 2017), which is the tradition, theory, and practice of interpretation and understanding in human contexts. The study involved a hermeneutic analysis of selected "suffering conversations" between family members and nurses. The selected segments of therapeutic conversations where suffering was specifically addressed was obtained from the Family Nursing Unit (Faculty of Nursing, University of Calgary) after the clinical sessions had been conducted and clinical videotapes were in the archived database. The chosen segments of the exemplary clinical conversations involving suffering were converted to audiotape and transcribed to text. The extracted segments of text were reviewed and analyzed by myself and other members of our research team in a hermeneutic process. The final results explicated the clinical descriptions and the exemplars of suffering were expanded into rich and full descriptions of the ways that conversations of suffering arise in clinical practice. It also illuminated which healing practices and interventions healthcare professionals offered within these therapeutic conversations contributed to softening suffering.

Below, I include two examples of my interpretive analysis of two transcribed clinical interviews. Hopefully, the reader can glean how useful the analysis and interpretation of particular conversations can be to uncover and reveal an in-depth understanding of suffering experiences of families who sought assistance and the identified interventions that softened suffering.

INTERPRETIVE MEMO #1

Uncovering Illness Suffering and a Way Out

Suffering seems to have completely filled the soul and mind of a young forty-year-old man experiencing a serious chronic illness/disability.

His illness has invited him to live in a "room" filled with suffering and, consequently, he experiences every corner, every nook and cranny of this room of suffering as he describes his life with illness. One of the corners of this suffering is social isolation. He offers the heartfelt and heart-wrenching comment that "during the day, I only talk to God." Most forty-year-old men find they have little time leftover in a day to talk to God, but this young man offers that God is the only one he talks during the day!

Depression is another corner of suffering that creeps into the room. But, the most pervasive, most difficult, most soul-depleting corner of his suffering is loneliness. "I find loneliness very hard," but he believes his conversations with the nurse and clinical nursing team help him "get the words out of his mouth." Is "getting the words out of his mouth" a way of getting some of the loneliness out of his soul and cells? This loneliness manifests itself on Sunday evenings as depression. "I have Sunday evening depression—because my wife is going back to work." And, then it is Monday morning suffering as he "wakes up to an empty house," missing his wife, that perhaps invites more pain and disability. He is consistent and persistent in expressing his loneliness with comments such as "loneliness is affecting me more and more." Perhaps the persistence is necessary until the nurse clinician is willing to enter this room of suffering with this young man. "Entering the room" would mean acknowledging the suffering, not just offering ways of getting out of the room quickly with well-meaning but premature solutions. It seems that the nurse and clinical team never closed the door to this room, to say, "Okay, tell me about this life of suffering, this life of loneliness, this life of depression." "What an incredible challenge for you or is it more of a tragedy?" "It seems like a tragedy to me." "How do you do it everyday?" "How do you make sense of it?" "Why you?" "Why do you think God has let this happen to you?" It seems that the door of the interview room was always open, in wait for the nurse and team to run through and escape the full encounter of suffering. He tries again to offer another way for the clinical team to understand his suffering by talking about the corner of grief. "Grief is a big part of my life."

Finally, he tries once more by telling a story about seeking information from others experiencing the social isolation that serious illness brings by asking the tough question to his sister(-in-law?), "What do you do all day?" Sadly, he received only a hollow answer. As nurses, we need to meet suffering in every corner of the room and world that a client or family experience before we offer a way out.

INTERPRETIVE MEMO #2

Out of Sync and Out of Life

In the third session with this loving and devoted couple, the clinical team learns more and more of how this couple is "out of sync" with their own lives and with the lives of their peers. Being "out of sync" seems to have them also living as if they are "out of life", particularly the life they had once known and planned. Is it not the missing of a former life or the missing of what one had hoped for in life, with or without a serious illness, that is part of deep suffering? After periods of deep suffering, our lives as we knew them are changed forever.

This couple's life has now changed forever and consequently has brought them into a space of intense suffering and sadness. However, it seems that as this couple reveals more and more of their suffering, the clinician was more and more inclined to stay within her own "head," rather than fully enter into the encounter of suffering. Although the questions from the clinician in the illness suffering conversations seemed useful and relevant, a connection to or validation of the depth of suffering was missing. Could it be that entering into the world of suffering of those who are ill is too intense, too foreign, or simply too painful? As the therapeutic conversation reveals more and more about the losses of their lives, does it become more difficult for the clinician to comprehend or even relate to this couple as she mirrors them in terms of their marital status? Or is the clinician fortunately deficient in matters of suffering in her own life?

Inherent in the experience of suffering is often the sense of being isolated or alone, a sense of being different or set apart. Being "set apart" in suffering seems to invite the clinician to set herself apart from the intense experience of suffering.

The husband states that in the last month, he has "never felt this level of grief" and "doesn't see it going away." To this response, the clinician offers the idea that illness affects all family members and explores with his wife how her husband's illness has affected her. But, the timing is off and the suffering of the young husband goes unacknowledged. However, a most useful phone-in from the supervisor from behind the one-way mirror refocuses the student to explore more about the "tough month," thus taking both the client and student to a deeper understanding of suffering.

The young husband's response to this inquiry became one of the most difficult illness conversations for me to listen to as a researcher and my reaction was without the benefit of an "up close and personal" encounter with this couple. But, the depth of the suffering penetrated right through the video screen and off the transcribed text of the interview. His litany contained suffering phrases were, "It's an ongoing battle that is never going to go away." "Is this what life is going to be? Sometimes you think you're going to have a nervous breakdown." "Being sick and being alone is a very ugly thing." "You have to lower your expectations of life just to survive." Going into the trenches of suffering is indeed "a very ugly thing."

However, the timing was not right for the student clinician to invoke the gut-wrenching litany from the husband's wife of her perceptions of her husband's losses.

"I'm sad for my husband, of what he has had taken away and he has perfected the dance of what he has left. Sad he can't have a normal life for a man his age. Sad we don't have the ability to do what couples our age do. Sad we won't have a child—a big chunk of life has been taken away; don't look forward to anything, so that you're not disappointed."

Now it is obvious and confirmed that serious illness has put this couple "out of sync" with their peers. What is typical in the lives of others won't be experienced by them. Even, sadly, that they are "out of life" with their previous hopes, dreams, and goals for the future. And, finally, and most sadly, they are also "out of sync" with each other as the husband states that he "has more fear of living than dying," whereas is wife states that she is "more afraid of losing him than anything else." This is raw and deep suffering.

How do we, as health providers, assist a couple in the depths of this kind of suffering? What can possibly be said or done to soften their deep suffering? One beginning effort is to acknowledge that suffering exists. The acknowledgment of the sufferers and their experience of suffering by healthcare providers can be a powerful starting point to begin understanding and healing. However, in this therapeutic narrative, an illness suffering conversation occurred without an overdose of acknowledging or empathizing. I have learned from this family and many, many others that acknowledging suffering must be done and done frequently, before any hope of healing or comfort can occur.

But, some comfort and hope for healing does come through the ideas, reflections, and offerings of the clinical team. They commend this family's love for each other and their compassion. They also speak the unspeakable (Wright & Bell, 2009) about the effect of this illness upon this couple's life and relationships. They validate that this couple is "out of sync" with others of their age, but that hopefully "talking is healing," and offers a unique and new idea for this couple about "making a space for living apart from illness from time to time… a place for illness, and a place NOT for illness." This idea captured this couple as the husband said, "Not even in our closets are we illness free." I would add that not even their closets are free from suffering. And, this young wife added that they had "no holiday last year or a break from illness." Another comment by the clinical supervisor to the family recognized that those who suffer with serious illness, loss, or disability need reassurance, hope, and above all that they are still cherished by others, especially their spouse, and even by themselves. The supervisor said, "Thank you for the gift we were privileged to listen to." This is a lovely example of reassuring this couple that their lives are still meaningful and cherished, even to healthcare providers.

What was offered to this couple was indeed providing hope, reassurance, and comfort. But, I believe what also needed to be said was repeated acknowledgement and validation of the level and depth of sadness and suffering that this illness has brought into their lives. Still, the question remains, what was it about this couple's suffering that inhibited the clinician and clinical team from acknowledging and validating their suffering with more explicitness and more emotion? I believe the avoidance of acknowledging this couple's suffering shows how very difficult it is to be a witness to suffering.

The therapeutic conversations about illness suffering between nurses and families in this study revealed particular understandings and interpretations that have the potential of inviting greater compassion and caring by nurses and other healthcare professionals. The understandings about suffering that emerged from this study that were most informative and enlightening were: 1) there is a loneliness in illness suffering; and 2) listening to the "cries of the wounded" compels a moral obligation to invite stories of illness suffering. Deep listening required avoiding the trap of trying to soften suffering too quickly and before it is fully understood.

The specific healing practices and interventions that were gleaned from this research are: 1) bringing forth the illness narrative of how a particular illness has affected their lives and relationships; 2) asking questions that open conversations about suffering; 3) listening to the illness narrative with astuteness to suffering; 4) acknowledging the suffering experience; 5) challenging any constraining beliefs that enhance the family's suffering; 6) strengthening the facilitating beliefs that soften suffering and invite hope and healing.

This specific research study about illness suffering and others conducted within the FNU have substantially added to our understanding of the experience of illness suffering and the interventions and healing practices that are most helpful to families. My colleagues and I have been disseminating our findings widely through the professional literature and numerous presentations at professional conferences, workshops, and lectures. However, the ultimate goal of any of our research projects was to improve the care of families suffering with serious illness that sought assistance at the FNU (Bell, 2015; Wright & Bell, 2009).

All the aforementioned studies of particular clinical practices and interventions are revealing and compelling about the healing aspect of bringing forth conversations of suffering (Bell, 2016). The particular research studies conducted within the FNU strongly suggest that it is not just a good thing or a nice thing to provide opportunities for families to have conversations about their suffering, but that it is necessary and imperative for hope and healing to occur.

PRESENTATIONS AND PUBLICATIONS ABOUT ILLNESS SUFFERING

All the research studies conducted within the FNU have substantially added to my understanding of the experience of illness suffering and the interventions and healing practices that are most helpful to families. My colleagues and I have been disseminating our findings widely through professional literature and numerous presentations at professional conferences, workshops, and lectures.

In our presentations and publications as healthcare professionals, we must truly honor those who suffer with illness and who graciously participate in our research studies. We can do this through our tone, affect, and manner in our presentations and publications, plus by showing congruence between the research findings and our response to them.

We must ensure that those who suffer from illness (patients/families) have not gone unheard. We can do this by acknowledging and affirming that we have been touched and softened by those who suffer. Research about how to comfort and heal those who are suffering must not matter just in the moment of a conference presentation or a professional publication. It must matter in our clinical practice; it must matter to who we are as healthcare professionals.

Research that addresses the ill, addresses suffering. Therefore, our research findings, conclusions, reflections, and discoveries must illuminate suffering and how to heal, provide hope, diminish, or soften suffering. Most importantly, our research findings must be offered in a manner that will be taken up in clinical practice. Hopefully, researchers who examine the interventions utilized with individuals and families will become more committed and attuned to the potential their research studies possess for healing. And, from the research process and findings, healthcare professionals in practice can utilize the ideas from the findings, plus add their own new ideas so we can reaffirm and reclaim our desire and motivation to be healers to those who suffer.

The dearth of scholarship about suffering in patient care is evidenced in the fact that major healthcare texts and bibliographical databases contain few citations about suffering. Reed (2003) suggests that those that do exist tend to equate suffering with physiological pain or to treat it as an indicator of disease or a secondary focus or illness. I concur that there is no agreed upon theory of suffering in the literature, nor any premises that lead to a consistent or common definition of suffering. However, it is my hope that this text will add one more voice to the efforts of healthcare professionals who do attempt to study, understand, and soften suffering. I trust that the most useful contribution of this chapter, and this book as a whole, is the actual clinical examples with individuals and families.

REFERENCES

Bell, J. M. (2015). Growing the science of Family Systems Nursing: Family health intervention research focused on illness suffering and family healing [L'avancement de la recherché sur l'intervention infirmiere systémique en santé familiale: bilan]. In F. Duhamel (Ed.), *La santé et la famille: Une approche systémique en soins infirmiers* [*Families and health: A systemic approach in nursing care*] (3rd ed., 102-125.) Montreal, Quebec, Canada: Gaëtan Morin editeur, Chenelière Éducation. [in French] English language translation available from U of C Institutional Repository, PRISM:http://hdl.handle.net/1880/51114.

Bell. J. M. (2008). The Family Nursing Unit, University of Calgary: Reflections on 25 years of clinical scholarship (1982-2007) and closure announcement [Editorial]. *Journal of Family Nursing, 14*(3), 275-288. doi: 10.1177/1074840708323598.

Chesla, C. (2005). Nursing science and chronic illness: Articulating suffering and possibility in family life. *Journal of Family Nursing, 11*(4), 371-387 DOI: 10.1177/1074840705281781.

Duhamel, F. (1994). A family systems approach: Three families with a hypertensive family member. *Family Systems Medicine, 12*(4), 391-404. doi: 10.1037/h0089166.

Duhamel, F., Watson, W. L., & Wright, L. M. (1994). A family systems nursing approach to hypertension. *Canadian Journal of Cardiovascular Nursing, 5*(4), 14-24. Retrieved from https://dspace.ucalgary.ca/handle/1880/44060.

Ehrenreich, B. (2009). *Smile or die: How positive thinking fooled America and the world.* London: Granta Books.

Ferrell, B.R. & Coyle, N. (2008). *The nature of suffering and the goals of nursing.* New York, NY: Oxford University Press.

Frank, A.W. (1994). Interrupted stories, interrupted lives. *Second Opinion, 20*(1), 11-18.

Frank, A. (1998). Just listening: Narrative and deep illness. *Families, Systems, and Health, 16*(3), 197-212.

Frank, A. (2001). Can we research suffering? *Qualitative Health Research, 11*(3), 353-362.

Gottlieb, L. (2007). A tribute to the Calgary Family Nursing Unit: Lessons that go beyond family nursing [Editorial]. *Canadian Journal of Nursing Research*, 39(3), 7-11.

Houger Limacher, L. (2003). *Commendations: The healing potential of one Family Systems Nursing intervention.* Unpublished doctoral thesis, University of Calgary, Alberta, Canada. Retrieved from http://dspace.ucalgary.ca/handle/1880/49062.

Houger Limacher, L., & Wright, L. M. (2006). Exploring the therapeutic family intervention of commendations: Insights from research. *Journal of Family Nursing, 12*, 307-331. doi:10.1177/1074840706291696.

Kleinman, D. (1988). *The illness narrative.* New York: Basic Books.

Lindbergh, A.M. (1973). *Hour of gold, Hour of lead: Diaries and letters of Anne Morrow Lindbergh, 1929-1932.*

McLeod, D. L. (2003). *Opening space for the spiritual: Therapeutic conversations with families living with serious illness.* Unpublished doctoral thesis, University of Calgary, Alberta, Canada. Retrieved from http://dspace.ucalgary.ca/handle/1880/45183.

McLeod, D. L., & Wright, L. M. (2008). Living the as-yet-unanswered: Spiritual care practices in Family Systems Nursing. *Journal of Family Nursing, 14*(1), 118-141. doi:10.1177/1074840707313339.

Morse, J. M. (2010). The praxis theory of suffering. In J. B. Butts & K. L. Rich (Eds.), *Philosophies and theories in advanced nursing practice* (Chapter 28). Sudbury, MA: Jones & Bartlett.

Moules, N.J. (2010). Invited editorial. How do you feel something when there is no word for it? Reflections on grief in Brazil - - Teaching, nursing, and research. *Revista da Escola de Enfermagem da USP (Journal of School of Nursing University of Sao Paulo), 44*(2), 243-249. *ISSN: 00806234.*

Moules, N. J. (2000). *Nursing on paper: The art and mystery of therapeutic letters in clinical work with families experiencing illness.* Unpublished doctoral thesis, University of Calgary, Alberta, Canada. Retrieved from http://dspace.ucalgary.ca/handle/1880/40483.

Moules, N.J. (2002). Nursing on paper: Therapeutic letters in nursing practice. *Nursing Inquiry, 9* (2), 104-113.

Moules, N. J. (2009). The past and future of therapeutic letters:

Family suffering and healing words. *Journal of Family Nursing, 15*(1), 102-111. doi:10.1177/1074840709332238.

Moules, N.J., McCaffrey, G., Field, J.C., & Laing, C.M. (2015). *Conducting hermeneutic research: From philosophy to practice.* New York, NY: Peter Lang.

Moules, N.J., Venturato, L., Laing, C.M. & Field, J.C. (2017). Is it really "yesterday's war"?: What Gadamer has to say about what gets counted. *Journal of Applied Hermeneutics, January,* 1-8.

Reed, F.C. (2003). *Suffering and illness: Insights for caregivers.* Philadelphia: FA Davis Co.

Robinson, C. A. (1998). Women, families, chronic illness, and nursing interventions: From burden to balance. *Journal of Family Nursing, 4*(3), 271- 290. doi:10.1177/107484079800400304.

Robinson, C. A., & Wright, L. M. (1995). Family nursing interventions: What families say makes a difference. *Journal of Family Nursing, 1*(3), 327-345. doi:10.1177/107484079500100306.

Sveinbjarnardottir, E. K., Svavarsdottir, E. K., & Wright, L. M. (2013). What are the benefits of a short therapeutic conversation intervention with acute psychiatric patients and their families? A controlled before and after study. *International Journal of Nursing Studies, 50*(5), 593-602.

Tapp, D. M. (2001). Conserving the vitality of suffering: Addressing family constraints to illness conversations. *Nursing Inquiry, 8*(4), 254-263. doi: 10.1046/j.1440-1800.2001.00118.x.

Tapp, D. M. (2004). Dilemmas of family support during cardiac recovery: Nagging as a gesture of support. *Western Journal of Nursing Research,* 26(5), 561-580. doi: 10.1177/0193945904265425.

Tapp, D. M. (1997). *Exploring therapeutic conversations between nurses and families experiencing ischemic heart disease.* Unpublished doctoral dissertation, University of Calgary, Alberta, Canada. Retrieved from https://dspace.ucalgary.ca/handle/1880/26879.

Tolle, E. (2005). *A new earth: Awakening to your life's purpose.* New York, NY: Dutton.

Tolle, E. (2003). *Stillness speaks.* Vancouver, Canada: Namaste Publishing and Novato, CA: New World Library.

Wacharasin, C. (2010). Families suffering with HIV/AIDS: What family nursing interventions are useful to promote healing? *Journal of Family Nursing,16*(3), 302-321. doi:10.1177/1074840710376774.

West, C. H. (2011). *Addressing illness suffering in childhood cancer: Exploring the beliefs of family members in therapeutic nursing conversations.* Unpublished doctoral thesis, University of Calgary, Alberta, Canada. Retrieved from http://dspace.ucalgary.ca/handle/1880/48765.

West, C. H., Bell, J. M., Woodgate, R. L., & Moules, N. L. (2015). Waiting to return to normal: An exploration of Family Systems intervention in childhood cancer. *Journal of Family Nursing, 21*(2) 261-294. doi:10.1177/1074840715576795.

Whitney, O.F. (1996). Suffering. *Improvement Era,* March, 210-212.

Wright, L.M. (2015). Eckhart Tolle's spiritual words of wisdom: Application to family nursing practice. *Journal of Family Nursing 21*(4) 503–507. doi: 10.1177/1074840715606244.

Wright, L. M. (1997). Suffering and spirituality: The soul of clinical work with families [Guest Editorial]. *Journal of Family Nursing, 3*(1), 3-14.

Wright, L.M. (2009). Spirituality, suffering and beliefs: The soul of healing with families. In F. Walsh (2nd Ed.). *Spiritual resources in family therapy* (pp.65-80). New York: Guilford Press.

Wright, L. M., & Leahey, M. (1999). Maximizing time, minimizing suffering: The 15-minute (or less) family interview. *Journal of Family Nursing, 5*, 259-273. doi:10.1177/107484079900500302.

Wright, L.M. (1997). Multiple sclerosis, beliefs, and families: Professional and personal stories of suffering and strength. In S. McDaniel, J. Hepworth, & W.J. Doherty (Eds.), *The shared experience of illness: Stories of patients. families, and their therapists* (pp.263-273). New York: Basic Books.

Wright, L.M., & Leahey, M. (2013). *Nurses and families: A guide to family assessment and intervention.* Philadelphia: F.A. Davis.

Wright, L.M., & Bell, J.M. (2009). *Beliefs and illness: A model for healing.* Calgary, AB: 4th Floor Press.

Chapter 3

Spirituality and Illness

A sad soul can kill you quicker than a germ.
John Steinbeck

We are not human beings having a spiritual experience. We are spiritual beings having a human experience.
Pierre Teilhard de Chardin

Religion is for people who are afraid of going to hell. Spirituality is for those who've already been there.
Vine Deloria Jr.

Deep suffering invites us into the spiritual domain, even if out of our awareness. A shift to and emphasis on spirituality is frequently the most profound response to intense suffering from serious illness. For most people, a spiritual awakening happens in this process. If healthcare professionals are to be helpful, we must acknowledge that mere words cannot give voice to suffering, but rather experiences of suffering are ultimately spiritual issues.

The experience of deep suffering often becomes transposed to one of spirituality as individuals/family members try to make meaning or sense out of their suffering and distress. These "dark nights of the soul" are for many an invitation to transformation. Deep suffering leads one into the spiritual domain as the big questions of life are faced (Wright, 1997; Wright & Bell, 2009). Questions such as "Why is my child so ill? I have not been a bad mother." "What did I do to deserve this illness?" or "Who will want to care for me now that I'm so disabled?" When patients and family members recognize that their lives have changed forever from a particular illness or loss and are able to stop wishing or wanting to go back to life as it was; stop blaming themselves or others for their current situation; let go of anger or sadness about what might have been, and no longer resist their current situation, but rather embrace or accept "what is" and the truth of this moment, transformation has begun! It starts with a separation and then an acceptance of what was and a more profound curiosity and interest of what their life might be now, more open, more expansive, suspending all judgment, and embracing the present. Where and how the transformation for each person will be experienced is unknown; it's our great privilege to not only witness suffering, but to also witness the transformation. As healthcare professionals, we create a context for healing, for finding peace despite illness or loss, without directing the transformation in any particular direction.

The capacity of healthcare professionals to witness stories of suffering in families is central to providing the context for transformation; it is frequently the genesis of healing. In working with individuals and families, helping professionals have an opportunity for illness healing by inviting and witnessing illness stories, within which a "domain of spirituality" is encountered. This journey into spirituality manifests itself in the offering of reverencing, compassion, and love between and among family members and their health care providers (Wright, 1999). It is inviting and witnessing of illness stories, the spirituality that is embedded in our lived experience of the world, that addresses both clinicians and patients/families.

Distinctions between Spirituality and Religion

The domains of religion and spirituality provide many rich and useful ideas about how to assist those experiencing deep suffering. However, to implement these ideas into clinical practice, it is important and helpful to make a distinction between religion, which is extrinsic, and spirituality, which is intrinsic. It has been my clinical experience that persons and families with serious illness cope better if there is an absence of spiritual suffering or distress. Spiritual suffering is usually the inability to invest in life with meaning and purpose. To find meaning in all major events that arise in our lives seems to be a basic human need. Meaning can be framed within the context of spiritual or religious beliefs, or through adherence to a particular ideological viewpoint, be it philosophical, psychological, or political. By being clear about our view of life and possessing facilitating beliefs about life, we are less threatened by unexpected or unusual experiences.

The challenge of healthcare providers in working with family members who are experiencing spiritual suffering is to avoid falling into the trap of offering ready answers or explanations about their serious illness or loss; we should instead listen, seek understanding, and be curious and compassionate. In so doing, one hopes that family members will discover their own meanings for illness and reasons for believing what they do about their illness. It is further hoped that the illness beliefs they adopt will assist them to soften their spiritual suffering (Wright & Bell, 2009). Unfortunately, there are some religious healers who attribute experiencing an illness or slowness in illness healing as a lack of spiritual purity in the patient or family members, or it is God's will. This illness belief is often used as an explanation for failures to heal or respond to treatment. Some practitioners in the field of holistic health, with its emphasis on mental control over physical states, and the importance of mind-body-spirit integration, have offered similar explanations for failures when they imbue positive thinking to the extreme. Persons whose physical or emotional symptoms do not improve are sometimes labeled with very unhelpful and disrespectful words such as "non-compliant" or "resistant to change" (Wright & Levac, 1992). This kind of language implies that the healthcare professional has more correct ideas for illness healing than the patient/family. Instead of using non-collaborative language and labels, healthcare professionals need to engage in collaborative and loving interactions with patients/families that are more aligned with spiritual care practices.

Congruence between spiritual and/or religious beliefs and one's behavior or operationalized beliefs results in a general sense of well-being and wholeness, whereas a lack of congruence frequently results in guilt or shame. I noted one delightful exception to this correlation when a ninety-year-old woman who was having trouble remembering past events explained how much she enjoyed learning and playing the game of bingo. "She doesn't remember that she doesn't believe in gambling," her granddaughter explained with a grin.

Illness begs answers to the big questions in life, and frequently spiritual or religious beliefs offer meaningful and comforting answers, as well as being an integral part of the healing process. Are healthcare providers prepared to aid family members in their search for the answers to the big questions? If healthcare providers are to be helpful, we must acknowledge that suffering and, often, the senselessness of it are ultimately spiritual issues.

Many agree that there are and need to be distinctions between religion and spirituality in healthcare, though for some they overlap. Definitions of religion in the professional literature offer much more coherence and agreement than definitions of spirituality. Spirituality often seems like a vague and unclear concept. But, perhaps the very problem with definitions of spirituality is that we reduce them to a concept that invites many contradictory definitions. Other authors blend or integrate spirituality and religion (Koenig, 2004; Koenig et al, 2008; Hubbel et al, 2006). I found the discussion by Thomas Mattus, a Benedictine monk, in conversation with Fritjof Capra and David Steindl – Rast (Capra, Steindl-Rast & Matus, 1991) offered some of the clearest thoughts about the relationship between religion and spirituality:

"You can have spirituality without religion, but you cannot have religion, authentic religion, without spirituality...So the priority belongs...to spirituality as experience, a direct knowledge of absolute Spirit in the here and now, and as praxis, a knowledge that transforms the way I live out my life in this world...Institutionalization is one of the consequences when an original spiritual experience is transformed into a religion... religion brings out the intellectual dimension of spirituality, when it seeks to understand and express the original experience in words and concepts; and then it brings out the social dimension, when it makes the experience a principle of life and action for a community. (pp. 12-13)

To consider religion and spirituality as *praxis,* transforming the living of life, highlights the relationship between them and may add a useful dimension to our understanding. In general, religion can be understood to be the language of the spiritual, which attempts to explain or describe the spiritual; spirituality itself *is* experience, according to the Benedictine monk Mattus. It has a language of its own that does not readily translate and is different from human language.

In addition to the formal conceptual models within nursing, much effort has gone into defining and conceptualizing spirituality as a phenomenon of interest. Nursing scholars assume that distinction, definition, and clarity will contribute to the integration of spiritual care in nursing practices. Spirituality is generally portrayed in the literature as a broader, more inclusive concept than religion (Wright & Bell, 2009; Wright & Leahey, 2013). Despite all the efforts in the healthcare literature, there remains confusion and lack of distinction between spiritualty and religion. Perhaps the struggle with clarity and definition may reflect the effort to study spirituality using the methods of the natural sciences, a predominant approach in the healthcare literature.

The foregoing discussion perhaps highlights the difficulties in resolving the ambiguity of both the terminology of, and the relationship between, spirituality and religion. Clearly there is a tension between the two that may be more important to attend to than to resolve through definition. The effort to differentiate terms seems motivated by the assumption that clarity will increase healthcare professionals' ability to integrate spirituality in their practices. This also reflects an interpretation of health professions such as nursing as an applied science, where theory is understood to direct practice. While some clarity is needed, too much may contribute to rigidity, a closing down, rather than an opening up of spirituality to understanding.

In summary, spirituality emphasizes the healing of the person, not just the disease. Healing is not curing, although a cure may also happen. And, a cure can happen without healing. Spirituality is not necessarily tied to any particular religious belief or tradition. Although culture and beliefs can play a part in spirituality, every person has their own unique experience of spirituality—it can be a personal experience for anyone, with or without a religious belief. Spirituality also highlights how connected we are to other people and the world.

DEFINITION OF SPIRITUALITY

With my previous thoughts offered about spirituality, I will offer my current definition that continues to evolve: Whatever or whoever gives ultimate meaning and purpose in one's life that invites connection, intimacy, and particular ways of being in the world towards others and oneself. It is being aligned with one's own inner being, spirit, or one's soul that is the seat of all inspiration, intuition, and wisdom.

The etymological roots of spirit include the Latin "pneuma," meaning soul, courage, vigor, and breath. Spirit is also derived from the Hebrew "ruach" and the Greek "pneuma," both of which also point to breath, or breath of life.

The terms spirit and soul, for some, have come to be used interchangeably, though within the healthcare literature the term "spirit" is used much more commonly. In other cases, soul continues to be interpreted as one aspect of spirit (Anderson, 2009). In this understanding, soul is tied to the body and mind, including thought, action, and emotion. Soul relates to the immanence, rather than the transcendence, of spirit.

A useful, modern definition of what spirituality is not is offered by Christine Hassler, the author of *Expectation Hangover* (2014). She suggests it is not about how much we meditate or how often we go to church or how many yoga poses or Sanskrit words we know. Or how much time we spend praying or how many Om pieces of jewelry we have. I agree. Yes, spirituality is not about our outward, observable behaviors and rituals that can be significant and meaningful within the context of most major religions. But, rather, spirituality is an internal, ongoing process of our evolving, reflecting lives and the sorting out of the meaning and purpose of experiences that come to us, and we to them. They invite constant revisions of ourselves and subsequently how we connect and respond to others, guided by our own spiritual wisdom, inspiration, and/or intuition. The stumbling block for a lot of healthcare professionals is that they conceptualize spirituality is either a religious belief or some kind of new-age belief, and they often don't know what to do with either one of those ideas. But, when healthcare professionals can broaden their idea or definition of spirituality and spiritual care practices to one of opening a sacred space for therapeutic conversations about illness suffering and illness healing, both patient and healthcare professionals are edified.

DEFINITION OF RELIGION

My current definition of religion is: The

affiliation or membership in a particular faith community who share a set of beliefs, rituals, morals, and sometimes a health code centered on a defined Higher or Transcendent Power most frequently referred to as God.

The great faith traditions of Buddhism, Islam, Hinduism, Judaism, and Christianity all have human suffering as their core. For example, the Buddha only understood suffering when he left his parents palatial home and witnessed suffering for the first time and came to understand that all life is suffering; Moses, as recorded in the Torah and the Old Testament of the Bible, who had all the benefits of being royalty and an Egyptian citizen, instead chose to suffer with his own people despite their slavery and oppression; Christian scholars have interpreted Biblical scriptures from the New Testament of the Bible that Jesus suffered even more in the Garden of Gethsemane than on the cross; Hinduism espouses that suffering arises if not enough good karma has been accumulated over a person's life; and, in Islam, it is a Muslim belief that suffering is due to one's own sins, and that to overcome this suffering, one must choose to do good. These very plain and stark examples of course do not do justice to the in-depth teachings and insights about suffering in these major religions. Rather, they are given to simply validate that all religions espouse human suffering as normal, and part of our shared humanity in the collective experience of "dark nights of the soul."

EVOLUTION OF SPIRITUALITY IN THE HEALTH CARE PROFESSIONS

Since I am most familiar with the history of spirituality in nursing, it will serve as the exemplar of the evolution of spirituality in the health professions. Interest in spirituality in nursing practices is not new, having existed as an integral part of nursing since before and after it's spiritual/religious founder Florence Nightingale (Dossey, 2009). However, over recent decades, there has been a resurgence of interest in the topic of spirituality on the part of theoreticians, researchers, and clinicians in nursing and other health disciplines such as psychotherapy and family therapy (Griffith & Griffith, 2002; Walsh, 2009); psychology (Nelson, 2009); social work (Crisp, 2010); medicine (Koenig, 2008; Puchalski, C. & Ferrell, B., 2010); and family nursing (Wright & Bell, 2009; Wright & Leahey, 2013). Although the interest has been significant, at least in the care of families, the deliberate inclusion of spiritual care practices remains a neglected aspect of clinical work (Wright & Bell, 2009).

Until the mid-20th century, nursing had been associated with, or actually existed under the auspices of, religious institutions. Nursing practice therefore has been strongly influenced by religious ideals, particularly an ethic of "doing good" and caring for those who are suffering.

Florence Nightingale, the mother of modern nursing, theorized about the spiritual focus of nursing practice. Nightingale believed she was "called" by God to serve humanity. To contribute to the development of a sense of spiritual well-being in her patients, Nightingale focused on developing "sympathy," a concept similar to the idea of empathy. Sympathy was understood as a mode for shared experience with others that included the idea of tolerance for others' beliefs and religious practices (Widerquist, 1992).

Gradually, however, as the natural sciences became the preferred way of understanding everything related to the body, nursing's spiritual and religious sensibilities became submerged in the Cartesian discourse that dominated the scientific curricula of nursing schools throughout the first half of the twentieth century. Secular views were separated from sacred morals, and physical reality from spiritual being. By the 1960s, illness was considered strictly a pathophysiologic event and the majority of nursing schools were no longer associated with religious institutions.

The overt religious commitments of nursing have been left behind, at least as far as the academic nursing discourse is concerned. The residues of nursing's religious sensibilities have been subsumed in the current topic of interest, spirituality. The nursing literature of the past few decades suggests that spiritual issues have been neglected in actual nursing practice, as well as in nursing theory and research. This acknowledgment seems to have sparked a renewed interest in the research and theory of spirituality and spiritual care, particularly regarding individuals, but also, to a lesser extent, with families (Wright & Bell, 2009). Far more of this literature has been centered in academic thought, while far less has been grounded in the actual practices of nurses, contributing to a proliferation of literature that has little meaning to clinicians and that provides little grounding for care.

The inclusion of nursing's responsibility for spiritual care cited by the International Council of Nurses, in their "Code of Ethics" (2012), speaks to the increased interest and reclaiming of spirituality in nursing. In addition, however, research on religious and spiritual topics has become more relevant in recent years with the burgeoning research evidence that spirituality and religion do make a positive difference in health and illness. The general public in North America has also demonstrated increasing interest in spirituality, though not particularly in traditional religious institutions, possibly adding further impetus to healthcare practitioners to consider the relevance of spirituality in healthcare.

Toward an Understanding of a Family Spirituality

One theme reflected in the theoretical literature is that relationships are an integral part of one's experience of spirituality. In some ways, then, it is strange that spirituality is taken up almost without exception in the professional literature as an individual phenomenon, with such limited acknowledgment of the social and environmental aspects. Perhaps this reflects the emphasis in healthcare to be strongly individualistic. However, if spirituality is understood to be about meaning-making that occurs in relationship and connection with others, family becomes key to both the experience and practice of spirituality (Tanyi, 2006). This is particularly so when one understands "family" as "a group of individuals who are bound by strong emotional ties, a sense of belonging, and a passion for being involved in one another's lives" (Wright & Bell, 2009). As Walsh (2009) has suggested, faith is inherently relational, from our earliest years, when the most fundamental convictions about life are shaped within caregiving relationships.

Religious and spiritual beliefs are among the most powerful beliefs we hold and contribute significantly to ways of making sense of the world (Wright & Bell, 2009). A core belief is understood to be a persisting set of premises about what is taken to be true and is forged in community, socially constructed in language within our families, and the larger community (Wright & Bell, 2009). Our beliefs are an ingredient in the glue of family and larger community.

Beliefs distinguish one person from another, yet also join people together. Through our living and being together, we influence each other's beliefs. We develop our identities within our families, professions, and communities through the belief systems that we share and do not share with others. We live our lives only slightly aware, and sometimes not at all aware, of our beliefs and the effect they have on our own lives and the lives of others (Wright & Bell, 2009, pg 20).

Family rituals are important avenues for the development, sharing, evolving, and passing on to future generations the belief systems that are of most importance to a family. Rituals are often religious in nature, including such things as weddings, funerals, and family prayer times. Family belief systems and their expression in ritual (both formal and elaborate; informal and simple) provides a way of making sense out of life events (Imber-Black, Roberts, & Whiting, 2003; Walsh, 2009), allowing us to preserve and enrich the spirituality embodied in relationships.

Anderson (2009) suggests that the renewal of an embodied family spirituality demands that we examine the metaphors that we use to think about the human person. The label of the *self* suggests a social construction whereas the idea of a person as a biopsychosocial spiritual being is more captured in the label *soul*. Soul thrives on a spirituality that is not only transcendent, but also grounded in the spirit of the family that is linked to generations of traditions, values, and stories. Stories are the memories of a family and a people, and it is memory that makes our lives personally meaningful by linking the past and the present. When we have lost our memory, we have also lost our soul (Anderson, 2009). Offering a place for families to tell their illness stories provides opportunities to claim memory and soul. Within the clinical practice of healthcare professionals, the inviting, listening to, and witnessing of illness stories provides a powerful validation of a profound human experience (Wright, 1997; Wright & Bell, 2009). Such validation might be understood as soul care.

WHAT'S LOVE GOT TO DO WITH SPIRITUALITY?

Is love not the essential ingredient within the relationship between patient/family/healthcare professional? Love is a powerful healer in the encounter of suffering. Nurses and other healthcare professionals can soften even deep suffering with love, compassion, and competence. But, what kind of love? I'm not talking about romantic love or even brotherly love. The kind of love I am referring to is love that opens space to the existence of another beside us in daily living. This definition of love is offered by the Chilean neurobiologist Drs. Humberto Maturana and Francesco Varela (1992). As healthcare professionals, it means suspending all judgment about our patient's/family's illness experience, their illness suffering, and their choices for illness healing/treatment options. It is what I prefer to call "curious compassion" (Wright, 2015).

The more curious we are about a patient/family's illness suffering, the more we can dissolve our own judgments and biases and practice in a space of curious compassion. It is in this sacred space that opportunities can arise for healing; that loving interactions can flourish. This is the kind of love to strive for in one's clinical practice with individuals/families. As healthcare professionals, we can open space for our clients and assist to them to unlock this basic emotion of love. We do so by becoming a particular kind of person in our therapeutic conversations, a person who is open to the ideas of others about their health/illness experiences; a person who does not blame/judge others' health/illness decisions; and a person who is open to having their own illness beliefs challenged (Wright & Bell, 2009). This kind of therapeutic conversation is one that consists of loving interactions, of opening space. No matter how sophisticated the technology of healing becomes, true healing involves love, that is, 'opening space' to others within a therapeutic conversation. Love is the invisible ingredient that is most significant in the overarching spiritual care practice of forming a healing relationship between patient/family/healthcare professional. For an actual demonstration of a family interview illustrating the healing power of love, I wrote/produced an educational DVD in 2016 entitled: *Therapeutic Conversations with Families: What's Love Got to Do With it?* (http://www.lorrainewright.com/lovedvd.htm).

THE RESEARCH LITERATURE: SPIRITUALITY AND ILLNESS

The favored language in nursing and nursing research is almost exclusively spirituality. This perhaps reflects the efforts in nursing to theorize about the nature of human beings and nursing's understanding of persons as biopsychosocial-spiritual beings to a much greater degree than some other disciplines.

Within nursing, research has focused on health-related outcomes, identification of spiritual needs with accompanying assessment and intervention, spiritual care practices, and interpretations of the lived experience of spirituality for persons and nurses. Although the language is more consistently about spirituality rather than religion, some studies do employ measures of religiosity. As might be expected in nursing, the health outcomes examined tend to emphasize issues related to illness, rather than disease, including such outcomes as coping and quality of life. However, with few exceptions, there has been very little research about spirituality in family nursing, family systems medicine, family psychology, and/or family therapy.

In the medical literature, which is largely American in origin, the preferred terminology, and focus of study, is "religion." This terminology is more reflective of the beliefs of American researchers, most of whom claim to be religious and identify more to the idea of "religion" than "spirituality." However, much of the literature has only looked at "religion," not spirituality, by measuring such variables as church affiliation and attendance (Koenig et al., 2001).

But, what about the impact of healthcare professionals' religious or spiritual beliefs on treatment? One study surveyed fifty therapists to examine the impact of their worldviews on their mental healthcare practices (Peteet, J.R. et al, 2016). Questions stressed worldview related to religion or spirituality, and how it was experienced in and influenced their practice and personal lives. The results indicated that, with regard to the influence of their worldview on their clinical practice, 19% indicated a great deal, 44% indicated moderately, and 37% said slightly or not at all. Most participants considered themselves religious and/or spiritual, although only 56% indicated a religious affiliation (37% said they were spiritual, but not religious). Researchers indicated that there was a "sea change" in therapists' worldviews toward religion/spirituality compared to surveys of psychologists twenty years before (both with regard to having a personal religious affiliation and being open to asking about clients' spiritual or religious beliefs). They also noted that there was a shift from affiliations being with traditional religions to orientations described as being "spiritual but not religious." These researchers concluded that differences in worldview may be associated with significant differences in ethical decision-making.

Family Health Outcomes and Spirituality

There is a substantial body of empirical research in the context of chronic and life-threatening illness that reveals a positive relationship between spiritual and religious variables and a wide variety of health-related outcomes. Some recent examples of studies examining the relationship between religious/spiritual variables and outcomes include coping with the loss of a family member (Walsh, 2009); and that family spirituality can assist in maintaining normalcy, cohesion, and resilience in the midst of crises (Boyd-Franklin & Lockwood, 2009).

Other studies indicate that families with strong spiritual orientations can effectively diminish family caregivers' burdens (Pierce 2001, Theis et al. 2003). Kloosterhouse and Ames' (2002) study further highlights that families' spiritual beliefs and practices can provide hope, meaning, and purpose in their lives when dealing with life stressors.

This body of literature is not without difficulties. Spiritual and religious variables for the most part are operationally defined and measured using existing instruments that are valid and reliable. However, many of the instruments have been criticized for not being culturally relevant for some and reflecting a strong Judeo-Christian bias. Although there are limitations, the findings across studies demonstrate the positive influence of spiritual and religious dimensions of life for health and well-being in the context of serious illness.

In addition to the empirical studies, there are accumulating numbers of studies guided by qualitative and interpretive approaches that also support the importance of spirituality in health and as a resource in illness and healing (McLeod, 2003; McLeod & Wright, 2008). One such qualitative study explored patient and healthcare providers' perspectives on the importance and efficacy of addressing spiritual issues within an interdisciplinary bone marrow transplant clinic (Sinclair et al, 2015). This study revealed, once again, that spiritual issues are a significant component of the patient experience, which when addressed may enhance patient well-being and satisfaction with care. Both patients and the healthcare providers stressed the need to address spiritual well-being in an open yet sensitive manner. While initiating and engaging in therapeutic conversations about spirituality sometimes elicited fear on the part of the healthcare providers, it was deemed a necessary aspect of comprehensive care that patients wanted addressed. One very interesting aspect of this study was that the experience of illness seemed to enhance *both* the patients' and healthcare providers' own sense of spiritual well-being. The researchers hypothesized that being in close proximity to mortality evoked a deepened appreciation for life not only for patients, but for their healthcare providers.

SPIRITUAL ASSESSMENT AND INTERVENTION

There is an emphasis on the identification or "assessment" of spiritual needs in both the theoretical and research literature (Borneman, Ferrel, & Puchalski 2010; Hodge, 2015; Tanyi, 2006). Spiritual needs are conceived of as the need to find meaning amid illness and suffering, the need for affirming relationships to self and others, plus the need for the realization of transcendent values such as hope and creativity, compassion, faith, peace, trust, courage, and love.

Research on spiritual needs clearly reflects a desire for theory that will allow control and prediction and a belief that once needs are clearly identified, nurses and other healthcare professionals will be able to intervene. This approach can invite rigid thinking or only the understanding of nursing as an applied science, or a technology. Conceiving of persons as a collection of needs oversimplifies complex human functioning and human relationships. Defining spirituality in terms of spiritual needs also invites a view of spirituality as a cluster of problems that by definition require a solution.

Nurses and other healthcare professionals vary in their ability to articulate the spiritual aspect of their practice. Just because some healthcare professionals may feel uncertain about spiritual care when asked does not mean that they are not providing spiritual care. But, I emphasize again, that it is the portal of deep suffering that brings healthcare professionals into the domain of spirituality. The spiritual domain for healthcare professionals is encountered by entering the "side door" or "back door," not usually through the "front door" in our therapeutic conversations with patients/families. However, religious leaders such as imams, ministers, priests, chaplains, and spiritual care counselors may go directly through the "front door" to inquire about spiritual issues.

Nurses can and do provide spiritual care that is embedded in other caring practices and these are, therefore, less visible and more tacit (see Chapter 5). Helping to make visible the unexpressed through studies of lived experience in practice may contribute to nurses' ability to articulate and ultimately strengthen spiritual care practices. Rogers & Wattis (2015) emphasize the importance that spiritual care practices should not be viewed as an invitation to share one's faith, nor an attempt to convert patients to a specific religious belief. And, I add to not pressure or even encourage patients/families to engage in particular religious practices, such as prayer. Inquiring if family members pray about their illness as a religious/ spiritual practice is very different than urging family members to pray. Religious practices, whether current or being brought forward when illness arises, need to come directly from patient/families, not from healthcare professionals. A spiritual approach involves opening conversations with patients/families to help them find hope, meaning, and purpose when experiencing deep suffering.

Some studies have sought to understand and identify nurses' perceptions of spirituality and spiritual care practices. One such study conducted by McSherry and Jamieson (2013) was very revealing. With a sample of size of 4,054 respondents in the United Kingdom, these researchers found that nurses struggled to conceptualize spirituality, even though they recognized it as being important to their patients. Almost 93% of the nurses surveyed believed spiritual care should be addressed, but only

5.3% felt able to meet the spiritual needs of their patients. Many more (3,688) believed they could occasionally address spiritual needs. However, it was not clear how they would do this, and lack of training in this area was evident. Santori (2010) also concludes that spirituality is an important aspect of patient care, but few nurses feel they meet patients' needs in this area. However, nurses tend to identify that "spiritual care" includes having a therapeutic presence, listening, and talking to patients. Interventions may also include referring patients/families to chaplains, clergy, or spiritual care counselors and providing religious materials.

Within our Family Nursing Unit (FNU), University of Calgary, the majority of studies were not specifically about spirituality, but it was uncovered that within therapeutic conversations with families, a discourse of suffering frequently opened up a discourse of spirituality (Wright & Bell, 2009). This points to the need to understand more about how it is that a discourse of spirituality is opened, is kept open, and what difference this makes to families.

Although not a formal inquiry, a clinical case analysis was done within the FNU of the ways in which nurses open space to spirituality. Four practices were identified in the therapeutic conversations between nurses and families (McLeod & Wright, 2001). These included (a) opening space for the gift of listening, (b) maintaining curiosity and openness to surprise, (c) inviting reflection on spiritual/religious beliefs, and (d) the invocation of metaphor.

A very enlightening study by McLeod's (2003) hermeneutic inquiry explored the meaning of spirituality and spiritual care practices as practiced in the FNU. She concluded from this study that spiritual care practices must include conversations about the meaning of illness in families' lives and relationships, and conversations about illness suffering and life experiences (McLeod & Wright, 2008). This study emphasized that illness suffering embodies an obligation to respond to the spiritual; to recognize that practices to create space for spiritual conversations include creating a sanctuary for stories of illness suffering to be heard; and the use of rituals in acknowledging the sacred. The results of these findings have been integrated to the spiritual care practices that I present in Chapter 5.

The need for spiritual care demonstrates that people are not merely physical bodies requiring mechanical fixing. People find that their spirituality helps them maintain health and cope with illnesses, traumas, losses and life transitions by integrating body, mind, and spirit. People, whether religious or not, share deep existential needs and concerns as they strive to make their lives meaningful and to maintain hope when illness, loss, or injury affect their lives.

THE RESEARCH LITERATURE: RELATIONSHIPS BETWEEN RELIGION AND HEALTH

Religiousness and spirituality associated with both mental and physical health is firmly established within the scientific literature (Koenig, 2008). In general, the effects tend to be positive, including lower levels of psychological distress and depressive symptoms, better health-related quality of life, and decreased morbidity and mortality.

A large body of research, mostly associated with disciplines other than nursing such as medicine and psychology, has focused on the relationship between religion and some health-related outcomes (Koenig, 2008). Although the language of "health outcomes" is used, many of the studies really examined "disease outcomes." Positive relationships between religion, often defined as church attendance and affiliation (though sometimes defined as spiritual well-being), and a wide variety of disease and health outcomes have been identified. In a meta-analysis of over 1,200 published studies on religion, spirituality and health, substantial evidence was found to support the idea that spiritual and religious beliefs are used to cope with illness and result in positive outcomes (Koenig et al, 2012). Religious beliefs have also been shown to be a positive influence on mental health outcomes such as suicidal behaviour, well-being, and substance misuse (Moreira-Almeida, 2006).

Epidemiological studies of mortality and

overall health, including some longitudinal studies, have documented these effects and both physical and mental diseases have been examined (Koenig et al, 2012). Examples of physical disease conditions that have been studied include cardiovascular disorders such as hypertension, coronary artery disease, and strokes, as well as cancer, immune system disorders, and a variety of symptoms such as disability and pain. In addition, relationships have also been studied with mental health disorders such as depression, anxiety, suicidality, substance abuse and schizophrenia. The consensus is that while many of the studies in the past were limited by homogeneous samples, cross-sectional designs, and inadequate measures of religious variables, more recent studies that overcome these limitations continue to show a positive relationship (Koenig, et al., 2012).

Koenig and colleagues (2001) suggest the need to examine possible negative effects of religion and also call for more longitudinal and intervention studies in a number of areas. The most pressing need they suggest, however, is related to the integration of knowledge into clinical practice. Religion predominantly has a positive effect on health, but it also has negative associations. Weaver and Koenig (2006) identified negative impacts such as delays in seeking medical treatment, guilt feelings, abuse by religious leaders, and religious factors often being part of psychosis. Feeling judged, criticized or shamed by a person's religious community can also have a negative impact on health.

Phelps (2009) argued that clinicians should consider patients' spiritual or religious beliefs whenever a poor or terminal prognosis is given. If there is deemed to be no value in treatment, preparing for death may challenge religious and/or spiritual beliefs. It may be appropriate to involve chaplains and spiritual care counselors if other healthcare professionals are not comfortable exploring religious/spiritual beliefs when a family is facing a life-threatening illness. These professionals may also help liaise with families in situations where patients cannot voice their opinions, such as intensive care.

The research trajectories proposed imply that knowledge will be integrated into practice through the eventual testing (using randomized controlled trials) of interventions that manipulate religious practices and experiences for the benefit of one's health once religious needs are determined. One example of taking a spiritual history is the CSI-MEMO. It is a five-item questionnaire to identify the following: Is religion a source of support and coping or a source of stress? Do you have religious beliefs that might conflict with medical decision-making? Do you have religious beliefs that belong to a faith community that might affect your compliance to these medical decisions? To what extent will your faith community be supportive? Are there any other spiritual needs that you'd like us to know about? (Koenig, 2011).

One of the most prolific quantitative researchers in this body of research, namely Harold Koenig (2008; 20ll), has clearly demonstrated the health benefits of religious practices, confirming the importance for healthcare professionals incorporating at least a knowledge and respect for this aspect of many patients and families into their practices.

However, what happens to one's health when people leave the religious faith of their youth and transition to no religious affiliation in adulthood? To answer this question, Fenelon and Danielsen (2016) analyzed data surveyed from 1973 through 2012, yielding a random sample of 34,565 adults in the USA. The religious dissatisfaction measure used in this study was developed by taking into account the religion in which the participant was raised and their current religious affiliation. In addition, researchers considered disaffiliation specific to the following denominations: evangelical Protestants, mainline Protestants, Catholics, Latter-Day Saints (Mormons), Jehovah's Witnesses, and Seventh-day Adventists. Health and well-being was compared between those who remained religious (consistently affiliated) and disaffiliates. The results indicated that disaffiliates experienced poorer physical health than the consistently affiliated. Similar relationships were present when comparing disaffiliates with the consistently unaffiliated and with converters. Relationships were mediated by frequency of religious attendance, since disaffiliates attended religious services less frequently. The effects of disaffiliation on poor health were especially strong in Latter Day Saints (Mormons), Jehovah Witnesses, and Seventh Day Adventists, and Evangelical Protestants; disaffiliation was also a particularly strong correlate of low happiness in Evangelical Protestants. This fascinating study, however, doesn't point the way to understanding what were the specific religious/spiritual beliefs that the participants held that could have correlated with their decreased physical health and happiness.

THE OBJECTIFICATION OF SPIRITUALITY

Objectification makes spirituality less recognizable, for spirituality always embodies a struggle in reaching beyond what is human to that which transcends our humanness. The development of "spiritual interventions" follows from the identification of "spiritual assessment," with both reflecting, at least to an extent, the objectification of spirituality as something that can be assessed and treated. This of course raises many questions, some of which have already been alluded. I have come to believe that spirituality cannot be 'assessed' or 'intervened' in this way. Questions of spirituality cannot be asked, answered, and recorded like we record a patient's temperature or fluid intake. Nor do I believe that it is reasonable to "intervene" directly in matters of spirituality if we embrace the notion that our primary and ethical aspiration as healthcare professionals is to soften deep suffering. Spiritual angst and distress can most often be assuaged and will be attended to when suffering is the primary focus.

What is clear from the review of current theory and research is that there are at least two fairly distinct voices about spiritual care practices that reflect certain epistemological assumptions and that have implications, in particular, for nursing practice. The quieter voice is articulating the lived experience of spirituality through the lens of suffering. Few of these studies, however, have explored spirituality as a practice in nursing care as did McLeod's (2003) study that examined issues of spirituality within therapeutic conversations (McLeod & Wright, 2008).

Far more prominent in the literature is the voice that, congruent with the natural science traditions, understands spirituality as an object, one that can be assessed, measured, quantified, and with which a nurse "intervenes." This standpoint is consistent with the literature in other disciplines investigating spirituality (religion) and health (Koenig, et al., 2001). Such an approach may be useful from an epidemiological perspective in validating the importance of spirituality and religion to health and illness. It is more difficult, however, to imagine how one will develop "interventions" based on the body of literature that will emerge from a research agenda informed by these understandings.

It is little wonder that some nurses and other healthcare professionals are uncomfortable with spiritual care when defined in ways of what is expected falls within a religious domain. Respecting religious practices and rituals with regards to health and illness is very different than offering spiritual care practices, such as those described in Chapter 5.

HOPES FOR THE FUTURE

There is clearly a need to understand more about the meaning of spirituality in clinical practice as it is lived. Nurses and other healthcare professionals continually address (and are addressed by) concerns and questions that can be considered spiritual and/or religious. Therefore, they need to become comfortable and understand that they are always in the domain of spirituality whenever deep suffering is addressed and know that there are specific and useful spiritual care practices that have the potential for hope and healing (see Chapter 5). Healing and hope usually happen in the slow lane as suffering is softened and spirituality awakened.

REFERENCES

Anderson, H. (2009). A spirituality for family living. In F. Walsh. *Spiritual resources in family therapy* (pp. 194 -211). New York, NY: The Guilford Press.

Borneman, T., Ferrell, B., & Puchalski, C.A. (2010). Evaluation of the FICA tool for spiritual assessment. *Journal of Pain Symptom Management 40(*2):163-73. doi: 10.1016/j.jpainsymman.2009.12.019.

Boyd-Franklin N. & Lockwood T.W. (2009). Spirituality and religion: Implications for psychotherapy with African American families. In *Spiritual Resources in Family Therapy* (Walsh F., ed.), Guilford, New York, pp. 76–103.

Capra, F., Steindl-Rast, D. & Mattus, T. (1991). *Belonging to the Universe: Explorations on the Frontiers of Science and Spirituality.* San Francisco: Harper.

Crisp, B. (2010). *Spirituality and Social Work.* New York: Routledge.

Dossey, B. (2009). *Florence Nightingale: Mystic, Visionary, Healer.* Philadelphia, PA: FA Davis.

Campbell, J. & Moyers, B. (1988). *The power of myth.* New York: Doubleday.

Frank, A. (1992). The pedagogy of suffering. *Theory & Psychology, 2* (4), 467-485.

Frank, A.W. (2000, April). *Can we research suffering?* Keynote address at the Sixth Annual Qualitative Health Research Conference, Banff, Alberta.

Frankl, V. E. (1962). *Man's search for meaning. (I. Lasch, Trans.).* Boston: Beacon.

Fenelon A, & Danielsen, S. (2016). Leaving my religion: understanding the relationship between religious disaffiliation, health, and well-being. *Social Science Research, 57*, 49-62.

Griffith, J.L. & Griffith, M.E. (2002). *Encountering the sacred in psychotherapy: How to talk with people about their spiritual lives.* New York: The Guilford Press.

Hassler, C. (2014). Expectation hangover: Overcoming disappointment, in work, love, and life. Novato, CA; New World Library.

Hoad, T. F. (Ed.). (1996). *The concise oxford dictionary of English etymology.* New York, NY: Oxford University Press.

Hodge, D.R. (2015). Administering a two-stage spiritual assessment in healthcare settings: A necessary component of ethical and effective care. *Journal of Nursing Management, 23*, 27-38.

Hubbell S.L., Woodard, E.K., Barksdale-Brown, D.J., Parker, J.S. (2006) Spiritual care practices of nurse practitioners in federally designated nonmetropolitan areas of North Carolina. *Journal of the American Academy of Nurse Practitioners. 18,* 8, 379-385.

Imber Black, E., Roberts, J, & Whiting, R.A. (2003, Revised Edition). *Rituals in families and family therapy.* New York, NY: Norton.

International Council of Nurses (2012) *The ICN Code of Ethics for Nurses.* tinyurl.com/n9redf9 Kloosterhouse, V. & Ames, B.D. (2002). Families' use of religion/ spirituality as a psychosocial resource. *Holistic Nursing Practice 16*(5), 61–76.

Koenig, H.G. (2008). *Medicine, religion, and health.* West Conshohocken, PA: Templeton Foundation Press.

Koenig, H.G. (2011). *Spirituality and health research: Methods, measure, statistics, and resources.* West Conshohocken, PA: Templeton Foundation Press.

Koenig H.G. (2004) Religion, spirituality, and medicine: research findings and implications for clinical practice. *Southern Medical Journal.* 97, 12, 1194-1200.

Koenig, H.G., King, D.E., & Carson, V.B. (2012) *Handbook of Religion and Health.2nd Ed.* Oxford: Oxford University Press.

Nelson, J.M. (2009). *Psychology, religion, and spirituality.* New York: Springer.

Maturana, H. R., & Varela, F. J. (1992). *The tree of knowledge: The biological roots of human understanding* (rev.ed.) (R. Paolucci, Trans.). Boston, MA: Shambhala.

McLeod, D. L. (2003). *Opening space for the spiritual: Therapeutic conversations with families living with serious illness.* Unpublished doctoral thesis, University of Calgary, Alberta, Canada. Retrieved from http://dspace.ucalgary.ca/handle/1880/45183.

McLeod, D., & Wright, L.M. (2001). Conversations of spirituality: Spirituality in family systems nursing – making the case with four clinical vignettes. *Journal of Family Nursing, 7*(4), 391-415. doi:10.1177/107484070100700405.

McLeod, D. L., & Wright, L. M. (2008). Living the as-yet-unanswered: Spiritual care practices in Family Systems Nursing. *Journal of Family Nursing, 14*(1), 118-141. doi:10.1177/1074840707313339.

McSherry, W, Jamieson, S (2013). The qualitative findings from an online survey investigating nurses' perceptions of spirituality and spiritual care. *Journal of Clinical Nursing.* 22, 21–22, 3170-3182.

Moreira-Almeida, A. (2006) Religiousness and mental health: a review. *Revista brasileira de psiquiatria*; 28: 242-250.

Peteet, J.R., Rodriguez, V.B., Herschkopf, M.D., McCarthy, A., Betts, J.,

Romo, S., Murphy, J.M. (2016). Does a therapist's world view matter? *Journal of Religion and Health 55*:1097-1106.

Phelps, A.C. (2009) Religious coping and use of intensive life-prolonging care near death in patients with advanced cancer. *Journal of American Medical Association*; 301: 11, 1140-1147.

Pierce L. (2001) Caring and experiences of spirituality by urban caregivers of people with stroke in African American families. *Qualitative Health Research 11*(3), 339–352.

Puchalski, C. & Ferrell, B. (2010). *Making healthcare whole: Integrating spirituality into patient care.* West Conshohocken, PA: Templeton Foundation Press.

Rogers, M. & Wattis, J. (2015). Spirituality in nursing practice. *Nursing Standard, 29* (39), 51-57.

Sartori, P. (2010). Spirituality 1: Should spirituality and religious beliefs be part of patient care? *Nursing Times 106*(28), 14-17.

Sinclair, S., McConnell, S., Raffin Bouchal, S., Ager, N., Booker, R., Enns, B., and Fung, T. (2015). Patient and healthcare perspectives on the importance and efficacy of addressing spiritual issues within an interdisciplinary bone marrow transplant clinic: a qualitative study. *BMJ Open 5*: doi: 10.1136/bmjopen-2015-009392.

Tanyi, R.M. (2006). Spirituality and family nursing: spiritual assessment and interventions. *Journal of Advanced Nursing 53*(3), 287–294.

Theis, S.L., Biordi D.L., Coeling H., Nalepka C. & Miller B. (2003) Spirituality in caregiving and care receiving. *Holistic Nursing Practice 17*(1), 48–55.

Walsh, F. (2009). Integrating spirituality in family therapy: Wellsprings for health, healing, and resilience. In F. Walsh (Ed.), *Spiritual resources in family therapy* (2nd ed., pp.

31-61). New York: Guilford Press.

Walsh, F. (2009). (Ed). *Spiritual resources in family therapy* (2nd ed). New York: Guilford Press.

Weaver, A.J, Koenig, H.G. (2006) Religion, spirituality, and their relevance to medicine: an update. Editorial. *American Family Physician*; 73: 8, 1336-1337.

Widerquist, J.G. (1992). The spirituality of Florence Nightingale. *Nursing Research, 41*(1), 49-55.

Wright, L. M. (2015). Brain science and illness beliefs: An unexpected explanation of the healing power of therapeutic conversations and the family interventions that matter. *Journal of Family Nursing, 21*(2), 186-205. doi:10.1177/1074840715575822.

Wright, L.M. (2015). Eckhart Tolle's spiritual words of wisdom: Application to family nursing practice. *Journal of Family Nursing 21*(4) 503–507. doi: 10.1177/1074840715606244.

Wright, L. M. (1997). Multiple sclerosis, beliefs and families: Professional and personal stories of suffering and strength. In S. McDaniel, J. Hepworth, & W.J. Doherty (Eds.), *The shared experience of illness: Stories of patients, families, and their therapists* (pp. 263-273). New York, NY: Basic Books.

Wright, L.M. (1997). Suffering and spirituality: The soul of clinical work with families [Guest Editorial]. *Journal of Family Nursing, 3*(1), 3-14. doi:10.1177/107484079700300101.

Wright, L.M. (2009). Spirituality, suffering and beliefs: The soul of healing with families. In F. Walsh (2nd Ed.). *Spiritual resources in family therapy* (pp.65-80). New York: Guilford Press.

Wright, L. M., & Bell, J. M. (2009). *Beliefs & illness: The model of healing.* Calgary, AB: 4th Floor Press.

Wright, L.M., & Leahey, M. (2013). *Nurses and families: A guide to family assessment and intervention* (6th ed.). Philadelphia, PA: F.A. Davis.

Wright, L.M., & Levac, A.M. (1992). The non-existence of non-compliant families: The influence of Humberto Maturana. *Journal of Advanced Nursing, 17*, 913-917. doi: 10.1111/j.1365-2648.1992.tb02018.x.

Chapter 4

The Trinity Model: Beliefs, Suffering, and Spirituality

"I didn't need to understand the hypostatic unity of the Trinity; I just needed to turn my life over to whoever came up with redwood trees."

Anne Lamott

I have had the privilege of engaging in hundreds of therapeutic conversations with individuals and family members about their illness experiences. These conversations invariably include family members' illness beliefs about their diagnosis, prognosis, etiology, treatment, and healing. They also involve descriptions of their suffering and the meaning (or not) they give to their suffering. Conversations about suffering open up the spiritual domain as individuals/families wrestle with coming to terms with illness suffering.

It has become impossible for me to think about spirituality without thinking about suffering and illness beliefs. And, I find it equally impossible to think about suffering without talking about spirituality and illness beliefs, and so on. These three concepts or notions are thoroughly intertwined and are closely related. However, I will initially discuss each of these concepts separately since language does constrict us from talking about each of them simultaneously.

Therefore, I offer the Trinity Model with the hope that it will provide healthcare professionals with a useful framework for thinking about the complex notions of spirituality, suffering, and beliefs. However, models cannot stand alone. They are built on a foundation of many worldviews, theories, premises, and assumptions that inform the models that arise. Models are more understandable and meaningful if the underlying theories are articulated and made known. Therefore, to comprehend and use the Trinity Model in clinical practice with individuals and families, it is important to know the theoretical assumptions underlying this model. Underlying theoretical assumptions of any model are important to state because they are the foundation of the way in which those models are operationalized. The three theoretical foundations and worldviews that inform the Trinity Model are postmodernism, systems theory (von Bertalanffy (1974), and a biology of cognition (Maturana & Varela, 1992). These three theoretical foundations can be read about in more depth by the original authors or in a condensed version in Wright and Leahey's 6th edition *of Nurses and Families: A Guide to Family Assessment and Intervention* (2013).

Models can be and are very useful for

healthcare professionals in their practice with individuals/families suffering with illness. Models are helpful ways to bring collections of ideas, concepts, and notions into our awareness. Without this awareness, our clinical practice can appear to be haphazard and not based on any useful or organized thinking.

Consequently, I conceptualize the Trinity Model as a theoretical model, which shows the interrelatedness and interconnection of three concepts: beliefs, suffering, and spirituality. It is at the confluence or intersection of these three concepts that life's meaning and purpose are queried, questioned, found, affirmed, and/or challenged (see Figure 1). All three of these concepts need to be inquired about, explored, and examined when caring for persons and families experiencing serious illness, disability, loss, or trauma.

Figure 1 TRINITY MODEL

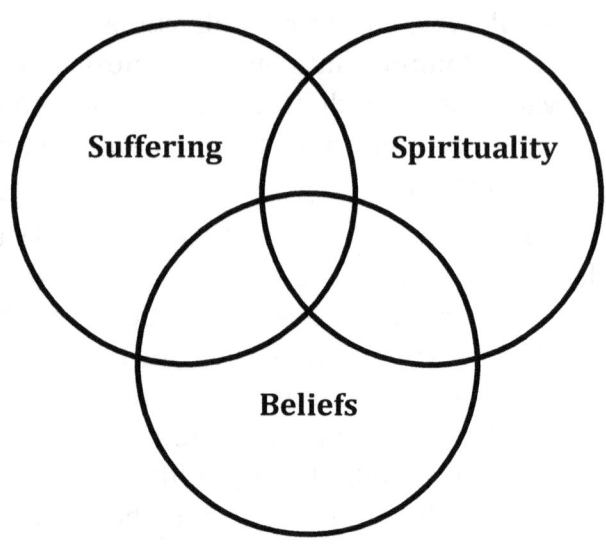

BELIEFS CONCEPT IN TRINITY MODEL

In our daily lives, the best medium for hearing our own and others' beliefs are within the stories we exchange in our conversations. Our beliefs are the blueprint from which we construct our lives and proceed to intermingle with the lives of others. At no time are family and individual beliefs more affirmed, challenged, or threatened than when serious illness emerges. What one believes about illness contributes dramatically to how one experiences an illness. No two people and no two families have the same experience with the same disease, whether it is the common cold or Multiple

Sclerosis. Some families view illness as a sign that they are sinful and disease as a punishment for ungodly living. Other families believe that being ill is a natural physical sign that the ill member should slow down and take care of him or herself, that no longer can his or her health be neglected. There are also many beliefs about how members should behave when illness enters a family.

Consequently, how families adapt, manage, and cope with illness arises from their beliefs about the illness that is confronting them. In fact, it is not a particular illness that may be a problem for a patient and his family, but rather their beliefs about the illness. Some individuals and family members cope very well with serious illness, while others do not. This is all related to their beliefs about the illness. What individuals and families believe about their illness significantly influences how they cope with their illness more than anything else.

The beliefs that family members hold are often reconstructed after the experience of illness (i.e. blueprints are revised); conversely, family member beliefs influence and shape the processes and outcomes of illness. For example, how family members treat even the common cold depends on their beliefs concerning how they "caught" the cold in the first place. If one believes that colds are related to experiences of stress, one will probably treat one's cold differently than if one believes a cold is due to inadequate rest and working long hours. If a person believes the best remedy for a cold is to rest, drinking plenty of fluid, and taking Vitamin C, that regime will probably be followed.

If the treatment remedy does not work, will the belief about the etiology of the illness be maintained? Will there be more openness to other treatment options when their original beliefs about the etiology and the cure of an illness have been challenged? Of course, there are circumstances when beliefs have little or no influence over the reaction of the body.

Not all beliefs matter to the experience of an illness. It is the core beliefs that I have found to be most useful to uncover and explore with families about their illness experience. Those core beliefs are: beliefs about etiology/cause of illness; beliefs about diagnosis of illness; beliefs about healing and treatment; beliefs about prognosis/outcome; beliefs about mastery/control and influence on illness; beliefs about the place of illness in our lives and relationships; beliefs about the role of family members; beliefs about the role of healthcare professionals; and beliefs about spirituality and religion and illness (Wright & Bell, 2009).

All healthcare professionals bring their own strong personal and professional illness beliefs to the clinical domain. Their beliefs influence how they view, assess, and, most importantly, care for and intervene with their patients and families. For example, a healthcare professional's beliefs about etiology may influence how a patient and their family are received, perceived, and treated. A healthcare professional who believes that obesity is a consequence of irresponsibility and personal weakness would likely respond differently to a family living with obesity than to a family living with the effects of a congenital heart defect, an illness over which a healthcare professional may believe the individual or family has no control. The core beliefs of healthcare professionals that will affect relationships with their patients and family members are their beliefs about illness, about families, about change, and about their own role as nurses in the lives of their patients and families.

Some beliefs are more useful than others in coping with illness. To uncover the beliefs that are useful and those that are not, a simple dichotomy of beliefs can be useful: constraining beliefs versus facilitating beliefs (Wright & Bell, 2009). Family members hold beliefs about their problems that are constraining or facilitating. Constraining beliefs perpetuate problems and restrict options for healing. Facilitating beliefs increase options for healing. Therefore, healthcare professionals need to focus on identifying and challenging, altering, or modifying family members' constraining beliefs about illness and draw forth, offer, and solidify more facilitating beliefs. The outcome is hopefully that the family experiences a new or renewed appreciation of their strengths and resources and increased options to discover and uncover solutions to their suffering. In the process, our own beliefs as clinicians are continuously altered and modified by our involvement with patients and families.

Dr. Janice Bell and I have substantially expanded and embellished upon these ideas about beliefs and illness in our text, *Beliefs & Illness: A Model for Healing* (2009). Therefore, I have only highlighted some of the aspects of the concept of beliefs in the context of illness in this chapter. The most important aspect to understand for the Trinity Model is to conceptualize the inter-relationship between beliefs, suffering, and spirituality.

CLINICAL PRACTICE EXAMPLE: "ARE YOU BEHIND IN YOUR LIFE?"

I now offer a clinical example of how exploring the illness beliefs of a young man opened space to his suffering and ultimately to a discourse of spirituality about the meaning and purpose of his life in the face of the impending death of his wife. Doran, a thirty-two-year-old married male, sought assistance from the Family Nursing Unit, University of Calgary (Bell, 2002) to assist him to cope with the impending loss of his wife to Lou Gehrig's disease (ALS). At the time of our clinical work with Doran, his wife Josanne, had been hospitalized for one year, was paralyzed, and incapable of verbal speech. Doran approached our outpatient clinic when his wife's anniversary date of hospitalization neared one year. Doran attended four sessions at the clinic, during which time he told the story of the impact of his wife's illness on his life. The following excerpts are from the actual clinical interviews that I was privileged to have with this young man.

Doran: I'm very, very depressed, Dr. Wright, you know, I'm really fighting a depression a lot.

LMW: Are you? How do you know you're depressed?

Doran: It's just that I don't feel good, I don't feel good most of the time. After our last meeting, I went and saw my family doctor.

LMW: Yes...?

Doran: Because of some major heart problems I'm having because of all the stress I'm under. And, I went to see him in the afternoon two weeks ago, and he listened to my chest, and I took a breathing test, right.

LMW: Yes...and?

Doran: And, he hooked me up to an EKG and he said everything seems to be okay. He said everything seems normal, he just feels what's happening to me, is my heart is, I'm under so much stress right now...

LMW: Right.

Doran: Smoking and drinking coffee and stress. He said I'm definitely experiencing, you know, symptoms related to that. And, he read my EKG and said there's no evidence of anything abnormal, right?

LMW: Umm...

Doran: But, I'm getting these palpitations every day and it's scary cause I'm just always scared I'm just going to (makes a sound here, like dropping dead), you know.

LMW: Are you?

Doran: I'm scared I'm going to die because of it, yeah!

LMW: Really?

Doran: Yeah!

LMW: When did you start having this idea?

Doran: Well, about, well I've been having these palpitations in my heart since November.

LMW: Yes, so are you saying that this is the scariest thing that you think about these days?

Doran: Well, it's everything...

LMW: It is the thought of yourself dying or is it the thought of Josanne dying that is the scariest? Which is the scariest thought? Yourself or Josanne?

Doran: Um... I don't know.

LMW: If you had to choose, which is the scarier thought, to think about yourself dying or think about Josanne dying?

Doran: That's a tough one, you know... I guess it would be the thought of me dying, you know. Um, knowing Josanne dies, I mean, it's going to be a relief, you know.

LMW: A relief for who, for Josanne, or for yourself?

Doran: For both of us? She won't be suffering anymore. And, I won't be suffering, neither will her mother, neither will anybody else that's got to go up there and see her like that, you know.

Comments: From this exploration, I learn how Doran's wife's illness is inviting him to suffer both physically and emotionally. He shares his belief that he is fighting a depression and that he sought out medical advice about his palpitations, but that no physical abnormalities were found. Both the physician and Doran believed that his palpitations were related to his present stressful situation of the serious, life-threatening illness of his wife.

But, much more was gleaned when I choose to "speak the unspeakable" (Wright & Bell, 2009), and explore Doran's beliefs about "Which is the scarier thought to think about, yourself dying or Josanne dying?" This question created an opportunity for Doran to offer his feelings about his wife's impending death. This type of conversation between myself and Doran opens space for suffering to be acknowledged and heard. It is during this part of the therapeutic conversation that Doran uses the word "suffering" for the first time by stating that "she won't be suffering anymore. I won't be suffering..." Now, we have a connection between his beliefs and his suffering. But, I suspect that this is only the surface of his suffering and I decide to gently explore the depths of his suffering.

LMW: I'm going to ask you what might seem like a really harsh, a hard question. I don't mean it to sound as harsh, okay as it may, Doran, but do you ever wish that she would die?

Doran: Yep (no hesitation). Yep, I wish that a lot.

LMW: Yes, because how would it make your life different?

Doran: How would it make my life different? I could go on with my life, I wouldn't be stuck like I am right now... I'm living a nightmare right now.

LMW: So, the anticipation of Josanne dying and the worry about yourself dying because of these heart palpitations, you are saying to me you feel you can't get on with your life, so if you can't get on with your life, ***are you behind in your life?*** Or is your life on hold?

Doran: My life is on hold, right now. Actually, I feel like I'm behind in my life... yes, I'm behind in my life.

You know, I feel like I have nothing to live for, you know. It's so hard, I don't know how long this whole mess is gong to carry on for, I don't know how many more months I'm going to have to go through this. I'm considering that I may not be strong enough to make it through the duration of my wife's illness and having to be out there and visiting her every day and trying to live two lives. I can't go on like that, that's the problem, you know, I don't know if I have the strength to go on.

Comments: The depth of this young man's suffering is now raw and exposed and has led me into a discourse of spirituality. He is questioning if he can live through this suffering or will he succumb to it by not being "strong enough." These conversations of suffering are indeed most difficult for me as a clinician, but I enter them because of my strong belief that if suffering is exposed, then possibilities for healing can arise. When suffering is submerged and not acknowledged, it festers like a wound that eats away at the very spirit of a person.

Once Doran shared that he cannot get on with his life while his wife is still living, this presents the opportunity for me to offer the notion that perhaps he may even believe that he is "***behind in his life.***" This metaphor seemed to fit perfectly for Doran as he repeated this phrase back to me. Now, we are entering the spiritual domain by discussing his meaning and the purpose of his life that invites him to behave in particular ways in the world towards himself and others. Through this therapeutic conversation, I learn that there is also spiritual suffering in addition to his emotional and physical suffering.

Because of Doran's frank admission that he has nothing to live for, I now have the ethical responsibility to ask about possible suicidal thoughts. So, I proceed.

LMW: Umm. Do you ever have thoughts of killing yourself?

Doran: Oh yeah.

LMW: How often do you entertain those ideas?

Doran: Well, I never really entertained those thoughts till lately and it seems to be more and more.

LMW: That those thoughts trouble you more?

Doran: Sort of, but I'm a Catholic and I don't believe in it. I've always been taught that if I take my life, I won't go to heaven, you know.

LMW: Ummm. So, do you think that this strong belief of yours will help you to get in the way or stop those thoughts of killing yourself?

Doran: I hope so, yeah.

LMW: I think that's a very good belief to have, isn't it? When you're troubled, it helps you to not take your life. Is there anything else, are there any other beliefs that you have that you think that will help you?

Doran: No.

Comments: The exploration of possible suicidal intentions leads to an important disclosure of his religious beliefs regarding suicide. I chose to highlight this facilitating belief as one way to challenge his constraining belief that there was nothing for him to live for. It was at this point, that I decided to validate his sadness and suffering, not about his wife's illness, but rather that he did not feel entitled to life.

LMW: Do you have any idea what I think about you at this moment?

Doran: I don't know.

LMW: What would you guess I think about you?

Doran: You feel sorry for me or whatever.

LMW: I don't think I feel as much sorry for you as I feel sad for you. Can I tell you why I feel sad for you? Would you be interested?

Doran: Yeah.

LMW: Okay. The reason that I feel sad for you is because I see at this point that you don't feel entitled to living.

Doran: Well, I want to live, I mean what's the point of living, you know, I mean I have nothing to look forward to right now?

LMW: Ah, so maybe it's a bit different then, so maybe you feel entitled to living, but it's trying to find a good, a good reason for living.

Doran: Yeah.

LMW: Because, at the moment, so much is focused on people dying. You are thinking about yourself perhaps dying, you are thinking about Josanne dying? Is that so?

Doran: I guess so.

LMW: Okay. Well, let me ask you a few questions around that. May I? Are you a person then that believes that you always have to be getting on with your life, or that you can never be behind in your life?

Doran: Yeah. Well, I've always been ahead in my life, but you know compared to most other people that I know, I'm behind in my life...

LMW: So, I'm trying to understand this, this is really important. If you were ahead in your life at one time, but now you feel you are behind in your life, do you think you're still a little ahead in terms of what you have accomplished in your life or are you falling far behind in your life right now?

Doran: Yeah, I don't have the things, like my sister's a year older than me and she's got, you know a lot going for her and other people I know who are the same age as me have a hell of a lot more going for them than I do.

LMW: And, a lot going for them in what sense? What's the biggest difference between then and you?

Doran: Well, they have their marriages, they have their homes, they have, you know, things like that? They've got really good jobs, and for the most part they have a very clear idea of what they want out of life, but in my case, you know, I just can't seem to get myself going.

LMW: Well, let me ask you, it sounds to me like one place where you are ahead in your life, that your friends are not, and your sister, is your sister married?

Doran: Yeah.

LMW: Yes, okay, one of the places that I see that it seems you are ahead in your life is that most young men your age have not had to face the anticipation of their spouse dying... they usually do that when they're much older...

Doran: Yeah, a lot of these men haven't had to face

that and they have really good jobs, they've got marriages, they've got a handle on what they want out of life.

LMW: Well, I'm wondering then, how is it that a young man like yourself, that is ahead of yourself in your life in one sense that you have to anticipate your spouse dying, way before most men do, but you are behind in your life in the sense of like you said, in terms of a job, being able to go forward with your marriage....But I'm trying to understand, how is it that you, Doran, have been given these challenges in life? How do you make sense of that?

Doran: I don't make sense of it....

Comments: Suffering tends to beg for explanation and the lack of understanding about our suffering seems to invite us to suffer more. In this clinical conversation with Doran, I am struck once again that the meaning (beliefs) we harbor in relation to our suffering can increase or decrease our anguish. Doran goes on.

Doran: I don't know, I try to figure it out and I can't figure it out, I just say, part of me just, when I think about that, right, part of me says, maybe if I was, I don't know.

LMW: Well, say more to me about that.

Doran: I say 'why me?'

LMW: Yes, 'why you?'

Doran: Why me? Why can't it happen to somebody else? Why does this have to happen to me?

LMW: And, why do you think?

Doran: I don't know. I don't have the answer to that?

LMW: So, you are sort of stuck in this question, 'why me' and not getting a satisfactory answer.

Doran: Yeah.

LMW: And, do you believe it's possible to get an answer to this question, or are some questions never answered?

Comments: The ever-frequent question of 'why me' is now plaguing Doran's mind. But, as one client so eloquently taught me, the question can be useful when reversed. 'Why NOT me? Why should I be spared suffering when others are not?' This is, of course, a very facilitating belief to the 'why me' question involved in suffering. And, Doran has his own facilitating belief that is now brought forth in conversation to help deal with his suffering.

Doran: Well, I believe that God's going to take care of me, you know, take care of my situation for me. I have to believe that.

LMW: Okay, so you believe that God will take care of you. Well, I think that's a very good belief to have.

Doran: Yeah?

LMW: Yes, and do you think this kind of belief could

make you suicide proof?

Doran: Yeah, it could.

Comments: Now, I link back to his thoughts of his life having no meaning and speak the unspeakable once again by asking if his beliefs could help to make him suicide proof. This unexpected context question is useful for bringing forth something which has been masked or lost. In this case, Doran was asked to bring forth his lost identity of being "suicide proof." I extended this line of questioning to sustain and distinguish more facilitating beliefs.

LMW: How else do you know that you are suicide proof?

Doran: Well, I've got people that really care about me that would be, that in spite of how things are, you know, I know that my mom and dad would always have their door wide open to me, right. If I ever had to go there...

LMW: Yes.

Doran: ... And stay with them for a few days there.

LMW: That's a wonderful thing to know, isn't it? Do you feel that's a wonderful thing to have that kind of backup?

Doran: Yeah, very much.

LMW: Okay, what other things make you suicide proof?

Doran: Well, I think the fact that I've spoken about it.

Suffering and Spirituality

LMW: So, the fact that you're even talking about it with me right now...

Doran: Yeah....

LMW: ... is another evidence that you're suicide proof.

Doran: Yeah, I think so.

LMW: Okay, that's very good. Anything else that makes you suicide proof?

Doran: I have things to live for, I have to believe that there's a better life for me, you know.

LMW: So, you believe that there's a better life! Well, that would certainly make a person suicide proof!

Doran: And, I guess another one is I'm getting help from different sources. I can come in here and I'm seeing a friend for coffee regularly and that helps, too.

Comments: In our four sessions with Doran, his emotional and spiritual suffering decreased dramatically as he brought forth more facilitating beliefs about his situation. Also, Doran and our clinical team were no longer worried about possible suicide as he continued to believe that his life had meaning and purpose in the moment, as well as in the future. Doran also began volunteering at the hospital where his wife was a patient, which was such a selfless way to give more meaning to his life. This was a young man who indeed was "ahead in his life" in several domains. This clinical example exemplifies how our beliefs can invite suffering and ultimately lead to questions of spirituality.

SUFFERING CONCEPT IN THE TRINITY MODEL

The alleviation of suffering has always been the cornerstone of caring. I believe that the ethical and obligatory goal of healthcare professionals, must be to soften suffering, be that emotional, physical, and/or spiritual suffering of patients' and their family members. All forms of caring aim in one way or another, to soften suffering. But, what is suffering? Much has been written about suffering in a variety of disciplines. My preferred way of conceptualizing or defining suffering is physical, emotional, or spiritual anguish, pain, or distress. Experiences of suffering can include: serious illness that alters one's life and relationships as one knew them; the forced exclusion from everyday life; the strain of trying to endure; longing to love or be loved; acute or chronic pain; conflict, anguish, or interference with love in relationships.

Individual beliefs of patients and family members are involved in both the experience of suffering and making inferences of suffering. Certain beliefs may conserve or maintain an illness; others may exacerbate symptoms; others diminish or soften suffering. Suffering begs for an explanation about why it has occurred and how it can be endured. Through the exploration of beliefs with patients and families, it is possible to understand how they are attempting to explain why they are suffering. When healthcare professionals can invite persons to reflect on their beliefs, those persons often become more open to considering other possibilities.

Suffering can reside within illness stories. From my own clinical practice and research with families, I have come to strongly believe that talking about one's experience with illness can soften suffering. To me, talking about, witnessing, and listening to illness stories in therapeutic conversations becomes the context from which suffering can first be acknowledged and then alleviated when healing begins. Telling stories of illness experiences invites the possibility of making sense of suffering. In short, talking is healing! (See Chapter 2 for further reflections about suffering and Chapter 5 for clinical guideposts that have proven useful to soften suffering).

SPIRITUALITY CONCEPT IN THE TRINITY MODEL

The influence of family members' spiritual and religious beliefs on their illness experiences has been one of the most neglected areas in individual and family clinical practice. However, there is much evidence that healthcare professionals are waking up to this neglected aspect of spirit in human experience. Increasing numbers of articles have appeared in professional journals, several books are now available addressing this topic, and healthcare conferences have more presenters offering their ideas about spirituality and spiritual care practices. This is an encouraging and needed development in the healthcare professions! (see Chapter 3 for a more in-depth discussion of spirituality in the context of illness).

My own clinical experience with individuals and families has taught me that the experience of suffering from illness, loss and/or disability becomes transposed to one of spirituality as family members try to make meaning out of their suffering and distress and find a path to healing.

The most significant learning about suffering that I have gained in my clinical work with individuals/families over forty years is that a discourse of suffering invariably opens a discourse of spirituality, if families and their healthcare professionals are open to it. Suffering invites and leads us into the spiritual domain. A shift to and emphasis on spirituality is frequently the most profound response to suffering from illness. If healthcare professionals are to be helpful, we must acknowledge that suffering and often the senselessness of it are ultimately spiritual issues Spiritual distress may be experienced by an ill person or family member who is questioning the reason for her or his suffering.

My preferred way to conceptualize or define spirituality is whatever or whoever gives ultimate meaning and purpose in one's life that invites particular ways of being and connecting in the world towards others, oneself, and the universe.

CLINICAL PRACTICE EXAMPLE: "WHERE WILL I GO AFTER I DIE?"

The proof is always in the pudding! The following clinical practice example illuminates the interrelatedness, and thus the trinity, of spirituality, suffering, and beliefs.

This family consists of a Caucasian sixty-three-year-old husband and his sixty-two-year-old wife. They have two grown children living in a different city. The husband had experienced a myocardial infarction six months prior to this session. The family had been seen for two sessions in an outpatient nursing clinic prior to being invited for a consultation. The couple had made good progress in their two sessions with the Master's nursing student and reported to me that talking about how the illness had impacted their marriage had helped to bring forth a lot of worries and fears that each were experiencing. Consequently, the couple reported that they were now talking more at home, having breakfast together for the first time in many years, and feeling more understood by each other.

When I work with families where one spouse has experienced a heart attack, I routinely ask the nonaffected partners if they worry about their spouses having another heart attack. I routinely do this as I have learned that this is one of the most common fears of a spouse of a coronary survivor. It was also the case with this couple and proved to be a critical exploration that opened even more alarming concerns. In this case, the wife responded, "Yes, all the time." When I asked the husband if he worried about having another coronary, he confirmed that he *does not worry* about dying from another heart attack. The most fascinating aspect of this therapeutic inquiry occurred when the wife disclosed her belief that *she* is going to have a heart attack! She also disclosed that she has been on antidepressant medication for twenty years because of her fear of dying. In the following verbatim transcript of my clinical work with this family, a significant distinction is made. (LMW indicates Dr. Lorraine M. Wright; W indicates wife; H indicates husband).

LMW: So, when you say (addresses wife) that you have a fear of dying, what do you mean by that?

W: I don't know where I'm going to go, that's the fear. I'm afraid. I don't know where I'm going to go, I don't know why. I mean I don't know if it's the religion, or the school, I mean it's the way I was brought up.

LMW: So, you're saying that the biggest worry around for you is not HOW you're going to die, is? But, where you're going to go AFTER you die?

W: Exactly.
LMW: I see.
W: Exactly.

Comments: This is a captivating and most important distinction and self-disclosure by this incredibly fearful woman. This dear woman clarifies that it's not the fear of dying that is most troublesome, but rather her fear of where she's going to go *after* she dies. Further clarification of her beliefs then ensues.

W: If you're good, then you're going to heaven, and if you're bad, you're going to hell. So, it was always on my mind, everything was a sin, so I grew up like that and I was afraid of everything and it's till on my mind today!

LMW: Hmmmm.

W: So, to me, I always see the clock (gestures a pendulum) and if you're good (gestures to one side) and if you're bad (gestures to the other side) and there's no middle. I don't know where I'm going to go.

LMW: So, when you evaluate your life today would you say…

W: Well, I was bad sometimes, like everybody else…

LMW: Sure….

W: But, then many times or most of the times, but uh….

LMW: But, when you evaluate your life now and you

look at your life, do you feel good about how you've lived your life?

W: Yes, sure....

LMW: Do you think, uh...

W: Sure, I wouldn't change my life, even though we went through a lot, I mean, with family and everything, but I wouldn't change my life anyway.

LMW: I wonder, I mean, I know quite a bit about Catholicism, but maybe you can help me more. Do you believe that you will be judged for the way you've lived your life here?

W: By God, you mean?

LMW: By God.

W: Exactly, yes.

LMW: And, so, if God were to judge you today, do you think He would be happy with you....

W: I don't know.

LMW: ... or not happy.

W: This is what I'm asking myself, you see.

LMW: AH... and what do you say to yourself?

W: We all know in my family I'm afraid to die, even my children. I kept telling them really so many times a month, I'm afraid, I'm afraid not to be sick or something, it's to die....

LMW: It's to die being fearful that you will be judged.

Comments: After this significant disclosure and further clarification of her religious and spiritual beliefs, I began challenging this constraining belief.

I attempt this by asking a question that I routinely ask in my practice: a hypothetical facilitating belief question (Wright & Bell, 2009). This question offers and embeds a facilitating belief and is an indirect way of challenging or altering a constraining belief. The question always begins with, "If you were to believe… " This question invites this woman to consider an alternative facilitating belief, one that suggests altering her beliefs may give rise to new stories and new behaviors.

LMW: This might seem like a very strange question, but I'm going to ask it anyway. If you were to believe, if you were to believe for even ten minutes today that God was very pleased with you, at how you've lived your life as a wife, as a mother, as a person…

W: That would change everything.

LMW: … what difference would that make in your life?

W: It would change everything for me.

LMW: Can you tell me what it would change? What would be a couple of things that would change for you?

W: First of all, I wouldn't be scared anymore, and then, I would say, well, if I die tomorrow; well, I die tomorrow, then I know where I would go. God knows when.

LMW: And, if you weren't scared anymore, how would you live your life differently, do you think? What would be different for you?

W: Well, I would be more, um, calm...

LMW: More calm...

W: Definitely, because it's all inside, it's working on me all the time and, uh, I wouldn't live that stress that I live all the time and... if you understand what I mean?

LMW: Yes, I do...if you could believe, I just want to make really sure I've got this—if you could believe even just for ten minutes that God was pleased with you, that you had lived a good life, that He would judge you very well, you said that would make all the difference in the world for you...

W: Exactly, yes, definitely.

LMW: ...that you would be more calm, and you would be more...

W: I wouldn't be on anybody's nerves like I am on account of death.

LMW: Yes, wow, that's incredible.

Comments: Here is a woman who has suffered terribly for many years with the belief that she will have a heart attack *and* an even more troubling belief that she doesn't know how she will be judged when she dies. Consequently, she does not know where she will go after death.

In this next interaction, an even more amazing revelation comes forth. This woman is now considering discontinuing all her antidepressant medication. Of course, this peaks my curiosity to learn if she were to believe she was going to heaven, would she need less medication? Her responses are astounding and her beliefs begin to change during our evolving therapeutic conversation. Her response is even more amazing as she completes my sentence and knows exactly the connection that I am hypothesizing.

LMW: I don't know, maybe this is a crazy idea, but I'm wondering, um, do you think that if you could believe that you were going to heaven, do you think there's any connection there; that you would need…

W: … less pills?

LMW: Yes, that you would need less pills.

W: Sure, definitely.

LMW: Wow! So, maybe this idea that if you have the courage, and are more positive…

W: Yes, just like a lightning (points to head, light bulb?), right?

LMW: You start think that "yes, I am a good person, I will, probably be judged very well, by God, and, be able to go to heaven." And I want you to know I have similar religious beliefs about heaven….

W: You do?

LMW: … and hell, and that we will be judged, and I hope I do okay, too, but I don't worry about it all the time like you do. That must be a terrible thing.

W: Oh, it IS terrible, sometimes I used to say to (her husband), it's terrible, you don't know what I feel inside, it's like I could scream.

LMW: Yes…

W: Some days I used to say, I would prefer to die, but still I said, I don't want to die.

LMW: So, you think there could be a connection there. So, as you would come off the pills, maybe then you would be getting more courage about believing more positively about yourself.

W: Exactly.

Comments: At the end of this session, I offer my impressions and commendations to this family. I offer what I believe that I have learned from this couple, particularly from this open, courageous woman. I also relate to her how I would like to tell her story to others.

LMW: I want to tell you a couple of my impressions and a couple of things that I've learned from you today! The first thing I have learned is that you've been married thirty-eight years, and the thing that you've really taught me today is that even after thirty-eight years of marriage, marriages can get better, it doesn't have to stay the same or get worse, right?

W and H: Yes, yes.

W: I'm so happy about that.

LMW: That you would probably say, I'm guessing, that

you would say your marriage is perhaps the best it has ever been, would you go that far?

W: Exactly, yes.

LMW: One of the best...

W: For me, yes.

LMW: ...one of the best periods in your marriage...

H: Oh, yes, one of the best periods for us.

LMW: ... periods in your marriage.

H and W: Definitely, yes.

LMW: See, that is incredible! After thirty-eight years, it's even getting better! This is one thing I've really learned today that we should never give up hope on marriages. That they can even get better, even after many, many years of marriage. The other thing that I've learned today that was very helpful to me is this notion that illness doesn't always have to be a terrible thing in a family. Illness sometimes can be scary, it can be a terrible thing, but some very good positive things can come out of it. Your marriage is stronger, you've come together, you've united more, and that's a very wonderful thing. (This occurred through their sessions at the outpatient nursing clinic). The other thing (addresses wife), when I go back to Calgary, my students will be asking me, "What did you learn?" I'm going to think about you, and you know the story I would like to tell, can I tell you?... is: the story about a woman who believed for many, many years, I feel very touched by this story... but, a woman who believed for many years that she was going to maybe be judged very harshly by God. That she wasn't sure if she would go to heaven or hell, and yet through her own courage she made a connection that maybe if she could give up this medication, there was a connection that maybe she didn't need to be on antidepressant medication anymore, if she could begin to have more ideas and better beliefs about herself. That she was a very good person and a good wife, and good mother. And, as she started to just THINK about that a little bit, and allow herself that idea, she also came up with the idea that maybe she could give up her antidepressant medication of twenty years!!! That is a remarkable story that I would like to tell!

Comments: As we said goodbye to one another, she told me that she had not wanted to come to the session that day, but was very grateful that she did. She spontaneously hugged me as we bid each other goodbye. And, I hugged her back.

As the therapeutic conversation evolved, I believe that we experienced increasing awe, respect, and a deep emotional and spiritual connection with one another. I trust that this piece of clinical work also illustrates the phenomenon of reverencing and love between this courageous woman and me.

Concluding Thoughts

The depth of one person's suffering is distinguished from others by each person's unique experience. I have ached, cried, and lamented when I have suffered with others, but it is only my own suffering that I have experienced firsthand. Suffering experiences cannot be compared, but unfortunately comparisons *are* made about which sufferings we believe are the most horrific. The most important role we have as healthcare professionals is to be listeners and witnesses to others' sufferings. We must acknowledge suffering; ask questions that will challenge any constraining beliefs that may be exacerbating suffering; and encourage more facilitating beliefs, possibilities, and opportunities for change, growth, and healing.

Through this type of exchange between family members and healthcare professionals about suffering, a domain of spirituality is encountered. This journey into spirituality manifests itself in the offering of reverencing, compassion, and love between and among family members and healthcare professionals. Likewise, these efforts to soften suffering cross the border into healing—a healing that is not reserved only for family members but also for professionals. Through highly privileged therapeutic conversations, spirituality, suffering, and illness beliefs become the trinity and the soul of healing in our clinical work with families. By healing is meant to live without suffering, to be at peace with one's illness or loss, and even to face one's death without fear. The Trinity Model can be a useful way to conceptualize the complex concepts and interconnections of beliefs, suffering, and spirituality within the context of serious illness.

Sections of this chapter have been reprinted with permission from *Spirituality, Suffering, and Beliefs: The Soul of Healing with Families* by L.M. Wright (2009) in Froma Walsh (2nd Ed.) Spiritual Resources in Family Therapy.

REFERENCES

Bell, J.M. (2002) 20th Anniversary of the Family Nursing Unit. *Journal of Family Nursing*, 8(3), 175-177.

Maturana, H., & Varela, F. (1992). *The tree of knowledge: The biological roots of human understanding.* Boston, MA: Shambhala Publications, Inc.

von Bertalanffy, L. (1974). General systems theory and psychiatry. In S. Arieti (Ed.), *American handbook of psychiatry* (pp. 1095-1117). New York: Basic Books.

Wright, L.M., & Leahey, M. (2013) 6th Ed. *Nurses and families: A guide to family assessment and intervention.* Philadelphia: FA Davis Co.

Wright, L.M., & Bell, J.M. (2009). *Beliefs and illness: A model for healing.* Calgary, AB: 4th Floor Press.

CHAPTER 5

Spiritual Care Practices

> *"Florence Nightingale who, by changing hospital conditions for victims of the Crimean War, brought about an absolute miracle. Perhaps no other woman, in the history of the world so far as I know, has done as much to reduce human misery, as this lady with the lamp, who walked through the vast wards of Scutari in the middle of the 19th century, spreading cheer and comfort, faith and hope, to those who writhed in pain. Hers was a life of excellence."*
> **Gordon B. Hinckley**

I wonder what kinds of therapeutic conversations Florence Nightingale engaged in as she nursed in those wards at Scutari with suffering soldiers who were wounded and/or dying. What in particular did she say that brought comfort, hope, and possible healing? What would we have identified as her spiritual care practices? We can speculate that with her great faith and her belief that nursing was indeed a calling from God that perhaps healing words or touch came easily to her. Or, perhaps she was more mortal than we know. Maybe even Florence Nightingale had moments of wondering what to say to a young twenty-year-old dying soldier worrying about the great suffering his death will bring to his mother, or another young man in great pain and suffering because of his shot off limbs. Nightingale writes "…the first idea I can recollect when I was a child was a desire to nurse the sick. My daydreams were all of hospitals and I visited them whenever I could" (Dossey, 2000). If her therapeutic conversations had been observed and/or recorded, I wonder what would be the same or similar to the spiritual care practices that I offer below. Through clinical practice and research, I have learned that effective and efficient therapeutic conversations *do* soften suffering and also invite and promote healing (Bell, 2016; Wright & Bell, 2009; Wright & Leahey, 2013).

This chapter offers spiritual care practices within therapeutic conversations (Bell, 2016) that offer possibilities for hope and healing. These spiritual care practices are exemplified by professional experiences, clinical vignettes, current research, and a detailed actual clinical example drawn from my own practice and research.

MACRO AND MICRO SPIRITUAL CARE PRACTICES

Over forty-plus years of clinical practice, I am convinced and dedicated to the notion that my primary goal and ethical obligation when working with individuals and families is to make efforts to soften their suffering. But, I emphasize that it is only through the portal of deep suffering that we actualize spiritual care practices. Through my extensive years of clinical practice and research, I have found the following spiritual care practices offer the greatest possibilities for healing: engaging suffering strangers; acknowledging suffering and the sufferer; bringing forth suffering markers; telling, listening to, and witnessing suffering; creating a healing context to soften suffering; inviting reflections about illness suffering; reverencing, loving and compassion; and challenging constraining beliefs about illness suffering. These spiritual care practices are by no means all-inclusive; they are simply the ones that I have found to be the most effective and efficient when encountering persons/families suffering deeply.

THE HEALTHCARE PROFESSIONAL-PATIENT/FAMILY RELATIONSHIP: THE PIVOTAL OVERARCHING SPIRITUAL PRACTICE

Nurses and all healthcare professionals make choices about the ways in which they position themselves in relation to patients and families. Such choices have implications for these relationships. Drawing on the philosopher Emmanuel Levinas, Frank (1992) suggested there is an inextricable relation between knowing the other, being known by the other, and knowing oneself.

If there is an objectification of spirituality, which can lead to measurements of "assessment" and "intervention," the relationship is often forgotten. When the relationship aspect within spiritual practice is forgotten, the healthcare professional's connection can become one of hierarchy, of "acting" upon, rather than one of respectful "being with." However, when the relationship is honoured and there is a desire to understand, acknowledge, and soften suffering, a spiritual practice emerges where patients and families feel "known." The establishing of the relationship can be considered the macro spiritual care practice, whereas the micro spiritual care practices are those outlined later in this chapter. In the following clinical example, this "knowing" by one particular nurse was perhaps out of her awareness, but was experienced as a deep relational, spiritual practice by the patient.

Clinical Practice Example: "Because she knows me."

Comments made by a family member during

a therapeutic conversation can often linger long after a meeting. This is usually experienced as a paradigm moment of learning for the nurse because the comments trigger an affective and physiological reaction and invite–deep reflection. Such was the case with a couple I had the privilege to meet and interview in Odense, Denmark. The husband made the comment during our therapeutic conversation that if he needed to speak to anyone about his health concerns, he would talk to his cardiac family nurse "because she knows me." The reason that this comment was so profound is that he had spent most of the interview espousing his illness belief that "talking" about his illness, his childhood, or any personal issue was not necessarily helpful or healing for him.

The interview took place at the 12th International Family Nursing Conference (IFNC12) held in Odense, Denmark in 2015, during a Pre-Conference Workshop offered by Dr. Janice Bell and me. The therapeutic conversation was observed live by a group of thirty nurse participants. Once the family meeting concluded and the family departed, we debriefed the session with our own reflections and those of the participants in the workshop. We also answered a few of the participants' questions about the clinician's intent during the interview. I conducted the interview while Dr. Bell led the pre-session discussion, reflecting team, and post-session discussion with the participants.

The couple being interviewed had generously agreed to participate in our pre-conference workshop and were recruited from the Heart Failure Outpatient Clinic in Odense, where they were involved in the Heart Failure Family Trial research project. The husband, Erik* was seventy-one with a cardiac condition, while his wife, Greta*, aged seventy, was experiencing several gynecological concerns. The couple had only been seen once at the Outpatient Clinic as Erik did not believe it was necessary that his wife attend these meetings with his cardiac family nurse Catrina*.

The family interview (therapeutic conversation) consisted of a short pre-session discussion where we shared the limited information we had about the family and invited the workshop participants to generate some hypotheses. This was followed by the actual therapeutic conversation between myself and the couple and the offering of a reflecting team intervention by Dr. Bell, myself, and four workshop participants. I then debriefed the session with the family and said good-bye to the family. Then, the workshop participants, Dr. Bell, and I offered our reflections in a post-session discussion.

The most profound moment of the entire family interview came during the conclusion. I had asked the family what stood out for them regarding the reflecting team's discussion and/or our entire therapeutic conversation. The husband responded:

"talking." This was a big surprise! For most of the time during our therapeutic conversation, Erik had related that "talking" was not necessarily healing or useful for him. But, then, he elaborated on his comment. He revealed a short narrative about his childhood and expanded on his previous comments of how he was deprived affection and love from his parents with poignant comments like "I was never hugged." However, he gave credit to his wife's family for embracing him within their family and enabling him to feel comfortable with family communication. This gentleman offered the notion that "talking" *can* be helpful as one of the insights he gleaned from our meeting when he had spent most of the interview defending his point of view that "talking" was not helpful.

Erik spontaneously offered the idea that if he needed to talk in the future, he would meet with the cardiac family nurse at the outpatient clinic who had been regularly meeting with him regarding his heart condition. Then, he offered the most powerful of statements about why he would feel comfortable talking with Catrina, his cardiac family nurse. *"Because she knows me."* Is this not the ultimate commendation for any nurse? Such a comment reflects the relationship that has been established—one of trust, compassion, and understanding without judgment. Was this not a spiritual practice to create this kind of trusting, compassionate relationship?

I admit that I had tears in my eyes at the end of the session as Erik disclosed more of his childhood story of deprivation of love and affection; how he gained some communication skills thanks to his in-laws, and then the remarkable comment of how he would confide in his nurse about health concerns, if need be, because she "knows me." This was a profound example of the healing potential of the nurse-patient relationship that opened a sacred space for this client. Indeed, this nurse was practicing within the spiritual domain, but perhaps wasn't even cognizant of such.

But, if we unpack the interview between this couple and me and identify some of my particular behaviors, coupled with the comments of the reflecting team, it is clear that there evolved a relationship consisting of a nonjudgmental and non-hierarchal stance. Particular interventions included: a more extensive exploration than usual of the husband's family of origin during the completion of the genogram because of clinician intuition; curious compassion of this couple's experiences with serious health concerns; acknowledging the husband's childhood suffering of deprivation of love and basic needs; resting from time to time on the positive about Erik and Greta's resilience and strength; and commendations offered by the clinical team and the clinician (Wright, 2015; Wright & Bell, 2009). This combination of relational practices brought about a touching and healing conversation for this couple; a marvelous and privileged learning experience for all who participated; and a profound commending of his cardiac nurse who "knows him." The evolving relationship between this couple and me, in just this one meeting together, became the most significant spiritual practice in this therapeutic conversation. As healers, we are involved in uncovering and nurturing, which I experienced and witnessed with this couple. The events of this therapeutic conversation remind me of the wisdom of T.S. Eliot who said, "We shall not cease from exploration, and the end of all of our exploring will be to arrive where we started and know the place for the first time."

*Erik, Greta, and Catrina are pseudonyms to honor the privacy of this couple and nurse.

Engaging with Suffering Strangers

Healthcare professionals are initially strangers to all the patients/families they meet. So, how do we as healthcare professionals treat strangers when we first encounter them? What are the essential ingredients to form a relationship that will enable therapeutic conversations of suffering to evolve? Surprisingly, I gleaned a renewed appreciation for this clinical skill when walking the Camino Frances for one week.

You may be wondering where exactly the

Camino Frances is and why people walk it. The Camino Frances is the most popular of all the Camino routes to Santiago de Compostela in Northwest Spain, the shrine of the apostle St. James in the Cathedral of Santiago de Compostela. Tradition has it that the remains of Saint James are buried there. Pilgrimages in the Middle Ages on the Camino were predominantly for religious reasons; while modern pilgrimages are less about religion and more about finding peace, seeking answers to tough questions; a time for reflection, thinking, healing, and for some simply the challenge of daily long distance walking.

For me, it was twofold: to have a unique experience for celebrating a milestone birthday (seventy years); and to provide a time of peaceful reflection while enjoying the challenge of daily long distance walking. But, the unexpected gift on the week's journey was my encounters with strangers and their kindnesses! A pattern of curiosity evolved with each new stranger about why each of us was walking the Camino. This curiosity was always met with a nonjudgmental attitude, and usually some act of kindness—from sharing food, to offering an encouragement that you *could* walk that last 6 km to the next village when you had already walked 20 km and were ready to quit.

Some of the strangers I encountered on my Camino walk were not seeking any particular healing or great epiphany. But, they all possessed an openness to whatever they might learn about themselves or others in their encounters with strangers. Other Camino walkers were definitely hoping for healing and/or trying to find answers to quell their suffering.

I was enlightened on this walking journey that the same ways of meeting strangers on the Camino were equally, if not more, important with those strangers experiencing serious illness. Kindness, curiosity, and non-judgmentalness needed to be in abundant supply with those experiencing serious illness, loss, or disability.

Is this not also true for the strangers we meet in our professional lives who become known to us as our patients and family members? Some are not seeking an answer as to why they are experiencing their illness, but are open to learning how to best cope or manage it. Others, however, are suffering deeply and cannot seem to find the answers to their questions of "why me?" or "why my family?" or "what am I supposed to learn from this illness?" In addition, do we as healthcare professionals have an open heart and mind to what *we* might learn from these new strangers in our lives, these new patients and their family members?

Another insight while walking the Camino was that because we were all walking in the same direction, we all arrived at the same village each night. The pace did not matter. Just as with illness, the pace of healing varies with each family, but the ultimate goal is the same... coming to a peaceful place with the illness; sometimes even giving up trying to understand why the illness arose in their lives, to become comfortable with not knowing.

Although there were times when I would walk a few hours alone on the Camino Francis, I also met and talked with strangers each day and experienced their kindness. For example, I marveled at the two young occupational therapists from Israel I met who had already grasped the relational aspect of families and illness. They loved to share their food while we talked. I was also grateful and delighted for the kindness of a young German man who played *Happy Birthday* on his harmonica to me.

But, it was Maria from Mexico who perhaps best exemplified the reciprocal nature of "stranger relationships" and the kindnesses that are exchanged. I met Maria on the Camino one day as we were walking along a particularly arduous ravine. Maria had come to the Camino with a goal to heal her broken heart. Her husband had left after twenty-six years of marriage and three children. He engaged in another relationship shortly after he moved out of the family home, but Maria wondered if this woman was the real reason he had left. Knowing of this "other woman" invited Maria to try harder to win her husband back. But, each of her efforts was met with a brick wall of cold and cruel behaviours and words. Rejection is a powerful invitation. I offered Maria the idea that resisting her situation (i.e. her husband was not going to return) was causing her to suffer more. As is often the case with those who suffer from a broken heart or an illness, she wondered why this had happened to her since she was "not a bad person." I left Maria with the mantra "stop resisting what is" (Wright, 2015). She liked this idea very much. I also offered her a commendation (Houger Limacher & Wright, 2006; Wright & Bell, 2009; Wright & Leahey, 2013). Specifically, I told Maria that I was incredibly impressed that she would travel all that way to the Camino to find healing; that it had taken courage to leave her family for a time and to focus on her own healing; and that I believed her healing had already begun because she was doing something different to resolve her suffering! Each step was part of her healing journey to begin to 'accept what is.'

While we were talking about her situation, we sat and rested on a couple of rocks. I had developed a pain in my leg that day and Maria just happened to have the perfect ointment for it. Kindness invites kindness. When we parted at the village of our final destination that day, we hugged and wished each other well.

I did not see Maria after that day, but I do believe it was not just coincidental that we met. Often, just as with our patients/families that we care for, we meet and care for those we need to care for and who need us.

In our clinical practice, we also heard stories of illness suffering and broken hearts. Just as with Maria, the very act of deep listening was healing, as well as the offering of new, facilitating beliefs and commendations (Wright & Bell, 2009). Patients/families help us to heal, too, when needed, if we are open to the notion that the kindness of strangers is a profound, relational experience.

A Biblical scripture seems to capture what might be the essence of the power and kindness of strangers. "Do not forget to entertain strangers, for by so doing some have unwittingly entertained angels."

Acknowledging Suffering and the Sufferer

To soften suffering it is of course essential to first acknowledge that suffering exists. Suffering is frequently the total sum of the illness experience, whether it is short and intense or prolonged and pervasive. Suffering is part of our human existence from stories of Job in the Judeo-Christian faith, to stories of holocaust victims, to stories of illness, disability, and loss. These stories belong to sufferers! The acknowledgment of being a sufferer and experiencing suffering by health providers can be a powerful starting point to begin understanding and healing. Comments such as "This time in your life is a really tough" or "It is a real tragedy what your family is experiencing" or "I can only imagine how difficult this must be for all of you" are examples of how to specifically acknowledge sufferers and their suffering. After acknowledging and validating one couple's experience with the suffering of a serious illness with their infant, the mother responded to me, "This is the first time that any healthcare professional has seemed to appreciate what a difficult and stressful time we have had. They talk to us as if life is normal, except you have an ill child. But, life is not normal and has not been normal for a long, long time." Another man when acknowledged about his suffering from leukemia said to me, "It is good to hear that you say we have been through a tough time because it has been very tough, but it really helps to know that someone else realizes that." These are only a couple of examples from the numerous times that families have responded in kind when being acknowledged that they are living in the mist of deep suffering. The deliberate and clear acknowledgment of suffering frequently opens the door for the disclosure of other fears or worries not previously expressed. For example, the fear of a caregiver who express the worry that if her health fails, then who will care for her spouse.

A profound personal experience of the healing that can occur when suffering and the sufferer are acknowledged occurred at the passing of my ninety-one-year-old father. It was a peaceful passing for which my family and I were so very grateful. Upon his admission to the hospital, we never expected it to be life-threatening or life-shortening. Of his brief six days in hospital, we had only two very hard, long days when my dad took a sudden turn for the worst. But, my family and I surrounded him with much love and caring and are confident that he knew of our presence during those final days and hours.

During his hospitalization, I was urgently called to return one evening as my father's condition had become life threatening. When I arrived at the hospital, the halls were eerily quiet at midnight as I rushed to my father's unit. He had been moved to a private room and a nurse and physician were waiting for me in the doorway.

They explained that my father's medical condition had seriously worsened and that they doubted he would "live through the night." I was comforted in that moment of how empathic these professionals' eyes were while delivering such staggering news. During my long night's vigil at my father's bedside, I also experienced nurses' empathic actions (e.g. bringing me a blanket and hot tea to ease the chill in the hospital room).

Miraculously, my father did not pass away that night. He thankfully waited until my brother/sister-in-law had returned from their vacation early the next morning. My Father gave them the blessing of being able to spend two more days with him.

On the final day of my father's life, the nurses who were caring for him showed continued compassion and empathy, both in their eyes and actions. Despite the healthcare professionals and our family knowing my father's life was rapidly diminishing, they continued to gently turn him; give him a sponge bath; and change the sheets on his bed. They explained to my father what their nursing actions would be, even though he had been non-responsive. These ever so kind nursing actions were deeply appreciated.

But, only one nurse was able to utter the compassionate words "I'm so sorry" to my family and me during those final hours. Could it be that empathic words require more courage and compassion than empathic eyes and actions? Are empathic *words* the ultimate acknowledgment of the suffering of others and a willingness to enter that suffering space? I believe so.

I am grateful for all expressions of empathy by those caring nurses and physicians on the last day of my father's life. But, it was those empathic words "I'm so sorry," not behaviors, that provided the greatest comfort to me on that day when the world changed. Those empathic words acknowledged me as a suffering daughter and those words were healing and have lingered as my grieving continues to unfold.

INVITING, LISTENING TO, AND WITNESSING STORIES OF ILLNESS SUFFERING

Talking is healing! (Bell, 2016) Inviting,

listening to, and witnessing illness stories of suffering provides a powerful validation of an important human experience. In so doing, we open the door to hope and healing. Healthcare professionals are in a privileged position to hear and affirm illness narratives. By inviting the telling of illness stories, we engage in the essential, ethical practice of recognizing the ill person as the "suffering other" (Frank, 2013). In my clinical practice, I also want to open possibilities, through therapeutic conversations, for recognizing the ill person and other family members as also the heroic other, the joyful other, the giving other, the receiving other, the compassionate other, the passionate other, and the strengthened other (Wright & Bell, 2009).

Positive responses from family members to spiritual care practices have persuaded me of the necessity to invite family members to tell their illness stories (Wright, 2007). In our professional encounters with families, we move beyond social conversations about the illness suffering to purposeful therapeutic conversations (Bell, 2016). I direct the conversation in a manner that I hope will give voice to the human experiences of suffering, as well as to the experiences of courage, hope, growth, and love. Through the telling of an illness story, the role of each healthcare professional is not only to be a listener, but also a witness to provide moral affirmation of the suffering that a patient/family encounters. Thus, the patient's voice must be encouraged, not cut off.

By providing a context for the sharing among family members of their illness experiences, intense emotions are legitimized. I have had many families tell me that having someone listen to their stories, ask questions about their stories, and commend them for their courage in the face of deep suffering has enabled them to gain a new and sometimes renewed appreciation of their ability to cope. Through this witnessing, listening, and commending, the family's resilience is often rediscovered with very positive outcomes (Walsh, 2016). In many instances, these positive outcomes have been the alleviation of physical symptoms and familial conflict, as well as to soften emotional and/or spiritual suffering. By inviting family members to share their illness narratives, which include stories of sickness and suffering, their own voices can be part of igniting hope and healing from within. Listening is hard, but it is a fundamental moral act.

Inherent in the experience of suffering is often the sense of being isolated or alone, a sense of being different or set apart. Such being 'set apart' in suffering seems to invite such conclusions, not only by friends and family, but also by the sufferer themselves. Our inclination is often to withdraw in the face of suffering, our own or others.

But, by inviting, listening to, and witnessing stories of suffering, we are not recoiling, retreating, or reneging on our obligation to listen to the voices of those that suffer deeply. So, how do we invite these stories of illness? It is through the asking of questions such as: "How has this illness changed your life?" or "I'm curious, what do you believe has been the reaction of your family members to your illness?" or "What has been the greatest surprise with your illness?" or "What has been the effect on your marriage, your children, of this illness?" or "What are you most concerned about with your illness?" These questions are invitations to hear and listen to how illness has affected individual and family lives. They provide opportunities for healthcare professionals to give the gift of deep listening and create a reverencing connection through the moral obligation to respond to suffering.

I have uncovered in my clinical practice that when a person is suffering, their internal conversations are usually filled with questions (Wright & Bell, 2009). To externalize these internalized conversations, I ask questions such as:

"What questions do you find yourself asking these days?"

"What questions do you ask on a good day/on a bad day?"

"Have you received an answer to these questions?"

"Do you need an answer?"

"What if you never receive an answer?"

These kinds of questions are entry points into the worlds of sufferers. Frequently, these internalized questions have not been spoken before and by externalizing them, clients report it begins to reduce the intensity of their suffering.

BRINGING FORTH SUFFERING MARKERS

Although there have been other illness experiences and deaths over the years with friends, friends' parents, and tragically even children, my most profound shaping experiences of suffering was the five-year ordeal of my mother's life as she, my father, other members of my family and I, dealt with the suffering and adversity of a cruel illness called Multiple Sclerosis. As my mother suffered, we as a family suffered with her. Initially, my mother's deep suffering was focused on her wonderment about why this had happened to her. What had caused this it? But, later, it was her physical suffering that took prominence, while emotionally and spiritually she became stronger. Even in her final year, when unable to walk or feed herself, she never lost hope or faith that perhaps one day she would walk again. Her tenacious and determined spirit lifted my spirits, initially.

My own suffering over those five years

took many forms: sadness, anger, anxiety, and even moments of great peace. There were many exacerbations with my mother's illness, each one leaving her more disabled than before. Thinking back on my own suffering that arose through the witnessing of my mother's debilitation, pain, and suffering— plus being acutely aware of the suffering of my father—there were particular markers that indicated my mother's life as she had known it was irreversible, and those illness markers deepened my suffering.

One such marker was a simple but powerful one, indicating the changes in my mother's ability to participate in her usual daily life. One such time was when I bought her first dress with Velcro strips. My mother, with her magnificent and plentiful wardrobe, was now in Velcro! I cried as I walked to my car following the purchase of her new Velcro dress.

Another major marker for me occurred in her finals days and weeks, when she stopped eating her meals. I knew this meant that the end of her life was near. For this reason, I needed her to eat. But, soon, we discovered that she loved the nutrient drink Boost and, for a time, that lifted my spirits as it seemed to keep death from the door. I would tease her that we would have to send her to Boost Anonymous as she was so addicted to that drink. On the day before my mother passed away, her marvelous caregiver was feeding her Smarties

(M&Ms). Smarties for breakfast! I was as happy and delighted to witness this unusual event as if she was enjoying a five-course meal.

Perhaps one of the most painful markers was the day I prayed that my mother would be released from her body, if that were God's will. I could not believe that I could utter such a prayer. I had listened to family members of clients over the years relate their pleadings in similar kinds of prayers. Yet, I could never, ever imagine having such a desire. But, there I was, wishing, thinking, and praying for the same thing. Whose suffering was I praying to release, my mother's or my own? In the final few days of my mother's life, watching her struggling to breathe in her tiny emaciated body, made me wish and pray for her death. And, just a few days later, she did pass away. Were my prayers answered or was it simply 'her time' or the failing of her body, or all of these? I do not know, and it does not matter now.

As my sister-in-law hugged my father and me at my mother's bedside at the time of her death, she uttered these comforting words: "Free at last." Yes, my mother was now free of this cruel, debilitating illness. And, we family members were also free of the unrelenting suffering of those five years. Free of the illness markers that had drip by drip enhanced my own suffering. But, of course, not free of the grieving that would begin. However, in the years since my mother's death, I have been amazed and surprised to learn, for me at least, that grieving was sweet compared to those years of deep suffering enhanced by markers.

The realization of how suffering can be enhanced by markers in my own personal experiences of illness with a family member have been usefully translated to my professional work with individuals/families. I now routinely ask family members questions such as "are there any markers or times when you realized that your suffering about your child's condition worsened because of a particular experience or event?" One young mother told me that one of the worst days of her child's chronic illness was when her daughter was not able to attend grade one as all her friends' children were doing. She said she had to stop looking at Facebook because there were too many photos of children on their first day of school, and she knew that her daughter's photo would not be posted. It was a painful marker, but she said that was the first time she had verbalized it. "Just saying this out loud, it feels like I can let go of it a little," she said.

CREATING A HEALING CONTEXT

The ultimate desired outcome is to create a healing context or environment for family members for the relief of suffering from their illness experiences. By healing is meant learning to live without fear, to be at peace with life, and to accept what is.

Healing is different from curing. Sometimes people heal physically, but they don't heal emotionally, or spiritually. And, sometimes, people heal emotionally, and they don't heal physically.

Eliciting, discussing, and expressing one's illness story and accompanying emotions can be very healing. Families have often remarked in my clinical practice how they appreciated the opportunity to talk about their illness experiences and the healing effect these conversations had on their lives and relationships.

One young man in his thirties was suffering with chronic pain experienced from Multiple Sclerosis. When I explored the deterioration in his MS since our last meeting, he told me he was experiencing much more severe pain in his chest and hands. But, as I invited him to reflect on his increased suffering, his beliefs about the treatment for this pain were fascinating. He did not believe that traditional medication was helping or alleviating his chronic pain. In fact, he reported that it made him "feel strange." Nor was he prepared to take any more steroid treatments. Rather, he told me that he had found some relief from his pain "by smoking an occasional joint." When I inquired about his beliefs about what he thought might be triggering these recent MS attacks and the subsequent increased suffering with pain, he believed it was due to the stress of his current divorce proceedings and having to move from his current home. He later told me that my question invited him for the first time to make this connection between his suffering from chronic pain and his divorce and this connection seemed to have a positive influence on reducing his chronic pain.

A dramatic example of creating a healing context occurred during an experience I had while travelling and lecturing internationally in Thailand. Three Thai colleagues/friends, a Canadian friend/colleague, and I visited Wat (temple) Kumpramong. In addition to the temple, the area also consists of a Center which functioned like a large palliative/hospice care facility, but with some stark differences from North American cancer care. The Center and Wat were located on a large expanse of beautiful, peaceful land, a far distance from any other towns in the Punnanakorn district in the province of Sakonnakor, Thailand.

The Center could accommodate fifty patients and their families who were experiencing cancer. No distinction was made between rich and poor families. All were welcomed, at no cost. The Temple and Center operated on generous donations from others. However, family members had to stay and provide the care to their loved one. A physician volunteered once or twice a week for medical assessments. Other volunteers also assisted at the temple for care and support.

The Center was led by a monk, Pra Ajarn

Paponpat Jiradhammo, who himself had experienced cancer. At the time that he fell ill with cancer, he had been a practicing engineer. But, life after cancer found him researching various healing methods that had led him to develop an herbal drink with eleven different ingredients. And that had led to his new vocation as a full-time monk. He was respectfully called 'Luang Ta' by the villagers. The herbal drink developed by the monk was one of the important interventions at the Center. However, in witnessing this intervention, I was struck by how many other interventions were embedded in that one ritual, and at the center as a whole.

Once a week, the monk offered prayers and an inspirational talk of Buddhist beliefs, wherein he would also offer hope and humor. Following his talk, each patient (or a family member if the patient is too ill) brought their package of herbal mixture developed by the monk and knelt respectfully in front of him. Prayers and a blessing for the herbal preparation was then offered by the monk. The monk also mentioned the name of each patient during the ritual.

Afterward, each family took the herbal preparation and immersed it in boiling water. Once stirred and boiled sufficiently, the drink was administered to the patient several times a day. The ritual was repeated each week. After this ritual, we had the privilege of meeting three families who had been admitted during the previous twenty-four hours. I was curious about what they were hoping for during their stay at the Center. All responded unanimously that they desired a "cure."

Later, as we walked about the grounds, we spontaneously encountered other patients and families who had been at the center much longer than a day; some for two weeks, others even two months. Very different responses were offered by these patients/families about their experience at the Cancer Center. Among those families who had been at the center for some time, amazingly, no one mentioned the desire to be "cured," but rather that they liked the peacefulness of the center, living with other families experiencing similar diagnoses, and helping one another.

One of our Thai colleagues arranged for a discussion with the monk at the end of our visit. During this discussion, I asked this very devoted and dedicated monk if the goal of the center was for "curing" or "healing." He offered that "patients/families come to the center hoping to be cured, but leave with healing; peace of mind and letting go of the desire for a cure. Indeed, some *are* cured, but the most precious outcome seems to be healing rather than curing."

The monk was also quick to offer that the herbal drink was simply but one aspect of the healing process at the center.

Leaving the Center, I was profoundly touched

by what I had witnessed and experienced. This Center combined many individual and family interventions that created a beautiful context for healing and softening suffering. Specifically, some of the interventions offered were: family support for an ill loved one and for other families; families forming a community of mutual assistance; spiritual wisdom from the head monk; and the ritual of praying over the herbal drink. This truly was a Center for cancer patients and their families that addressed the biopsychosocial-spiritual needs.

It struck me that the monk also functioned as a very wise and self-trained "healthcare professional." He was insightful and knew that when patients and families altered their illness beliefs and desires for a cure, their suffering softened and healing began. Is not the ultimate goal of all healthcare professionals to create a context of caring where healing may emerge whether or not a cure happens?

INVITING REFLECTIONS ABOUT ILLNESS SUFFERING

To alter existing illness beliefs, healthcare professionals need to invite family members to a reflection about their constraining beliefs (Wright & Bell, 2009). Through these reflections, a person begins to entertain different or alternative beliefs in order to get out of a state of confusion, struggle, or suffering. For example, beliefs about hope and optimism in the illness experience have generally not been addressed by the dominant medical system. Consequently, the appeal of complementary, integrative, or alternative healing approaches becomes very understandable. Many persons suffering with illness find these approaches more positive than the conventional medical approach because the complementary healing approaches do not shy away from some of the big questions surrounding illness: Why has this illness happened to me? Why do people get sick despite living well? Why do some people die "before their time?" Why is my condition becoming worse?

Another woman who was seen in the Family Nursing Unit was facing a double tragedy. Both her husband and young ten-year-old son had life-threatening illnesses. When asked about the impact of this on her life, she responded, "I myself am not afraid to die, I am afraid of living. How can I go on without the two people whom I love the most?" Through reflection, it is of course the ultimate goal that individuals and family members will find other ways to understand their suffering, to make meaning from their suffering, and ultimately to regain hope and resilience for their futures. This courageous woman found meaning in her faith, albeit that it was fragile for a time, to find meaning in her suffering.

We can also learn and invite reflections about various client and family members' spiritual and religious beliefs that may or may not contribute to their suffering. For example, a healthcare professional might inquire: "What are the beliefs of your Muslim (or Sufi, Buddhist, North American native, Judaism, or Christian) faith that help or hinder your suffering right now? What do Muslims believe is the reason for suffering? Do you agree with that belief? Has your experience with your illness strengthened or challenged that belief?"

Clinical Practice Example: "A Problem of Loving too Much."

I learned another valuable lesson while interviewing a couple in Japan about their illness suffering. Loving too much can make you ill. This lovely couple graciously agreed to a family interview as part of a teaching/learning experience I offered at Kitasato University. Dr Nami Kobayashi provided excellent translation for the family and me. Her knowledge of family assessment and intervention and familiarity with the models that I utilize when interviewing families was essential for competent and compassionate translation.

What was initially most striking to me were the differences in the physical appearances of this couple. Nori, a forty-five-year-old rehabilitation physician, was permanently disabled due to treatment of a cancerous condition of one hip. Consequently, he had been confined to a wheelchair for some fifteen years.

Despite a more recent and very troubling diagnosis and treatment of a brain tumor, Nori looked strong and robust with full cheeks; dressed immaculately in his suit and tie; and very attentive during the interview. His forty-six-year-old wife Hiroko presented a stark contrast. Although not disabled in her walking ability, she looked more "disabled" in her physical appearance than her wheelchair-bound husband. Hiroko was frighteningly thin, pencil thin, with eyes that appeared vacant. She sat still during the family interview, looking straight ahead, very intently.

What was evident was what I have experienced with numerous couples and families—that the person with the illness diagnosis is often not the person suffering the most. It certainly appeared that it was Hiroko who was experiencing the most anguish.

As the therapeutic conversation unfolded, I learned more details about this couple's illness narrative. I inquired about the impact of illness on their lives and relationships, especially their marriage. I also explored some of their illness beliefs about their current situation.

This couple had been married eight years at the time of Nori's frightening diagnosis of a brain tumor. Hiroko claimed it was like a "nightmare" for her. This metaphor captured well her past and current torment and suffering about her husband's condition. She reported that she worried about his condition 70% of the time and was anxious about whether it would "come back." Her excessive anxiety and worry had resulted in loss of appetite, sleep and even needing to live with her in-laws for a time to be taken care of when Nori was hospitalized for his condition. She also contained her worry and did not share her concerns even with her own parents. Hiroko did all the worrying for this couple as Nori surprisingly claimed he did not think about his condition at all; he was "busy enjoying his work."

The impact of the illness upon their marriage revealed that Hiroko has now taken on much more responsibility overseeing finances and completing their taxes. She also made a very touching comment that since they did not have children, Nori's illness gave her an opportunity to "protect someone." However, the protection of her husband had sadly evolved to erasing her own needs and aspirations.

As I normally do at the end of an interview, I offered this couple some commendations and recommendations. I offered Hiroko my conceptualization that she had a problem of "loving her husband so much that she had made herself ill." But, first, I commended Hiroko for the love, caregiving, and devotion to her husband. However, I suggested that it would be helpful in the future if she could find a way to love and care for her husband in a more "healthy" way.

By offering new and alternate views of her devoted caregiving, I invited Hiroko to entertain others ways she might care for her husband that were not at the expense of her own health. It was gratifying that she asked me shortly after my commendations and alternate illness beliefs how she might deal with her feelings of worry and anxiety. I was pleased with Hiroko's questions as they focused on self-care.

Since Hiroko had been erasing herself as a woman and wife in the world, I encouraged activities that would focus on her and her current health problem. One recommendation I made was that she learn meditation, as I explained it is often very helpful to persons suffering with anxiety. I also suggested she might seek out a cognitive behavioral therapist as another method of learning ways of gaining more control over the influence of anxiety in her life.

Since her husband, Nori, gained much support, love, and attention from his wife, I believed that shifting their couple dynamic from being less unidirectional (Hiroko to Nori) to more interactional would enrich the marriage and enable Nori to show more of his love for his wife. His love shone through when he asked, "what can I do for my wife?" This indicated that he too had reflected on my comments about his wife "loving too much." I asked him if he would be willing to take the leadership to inject more "fun" back into their marriage. I had learned that their only outings together were to attend conferences where Nori would speak about his condition and of course he would again be the focus of attention. They both appeared delighted with this suggestion and Nori said he would be willing to take the "leadership for fun" in their marriage.

Of course, it would have been easy to pathologize this couple (or any couple for that matter), but I prefer to be a strengths detective and uncover the competencies, strengths, and resources within couples and families and offer them commendations. The therapeutic intervention of "commendations" (Houger Limacher, & Wright, 2006; Wright & Bell, 2009) has the ability to invite family healing due to a new way for the couple to view their relationship with one another and their relationship with illness.

In a brief follow-up phone call the next day by one of my colleagues, Nori reported being pleased and satisfied with the interview, while Hiroko reported that she was "uplifted!"

Perhaps the more specific lesson learned from this couple is that erasing oneself to love another, even a loved one who is ill, is perhaps not love at all, but rather a prescription to make oneself ill. Simultaneously loving oneself *and* loving one's partner in a marriage enables both to grow, mature, and thrive. By offering Hiroko and Nori different and alternative illness beliefs about their illness suffering, it invited them to reflect in ways that have enabled their suffering to be softened and entertain new ways of being with one another. It was a privilege to have met them. I was very grateful to my colleague and friend Dr. Nami Kobayashi for providing the translation during this family interview.

REVERENCING, LOVING, AND COMPASSION

I have had one recurring piece of feedback about my clinical work with families' that has guided me in becoming more cognizant and appreciative of the spiritual dimension of therapeutic conversations. Colleagues and students alike have offered their unsolicited observations on the "spiritual" aspects of my clinical work for many years. I found this observation fascinating, as I had not previously put any direct or intended emphasis about spiritual issues in my clinical work. I reflected that, somehow, I must have changed from my early years as a clinician, as this feedback was news of a difference. The greatest reflection came following a valued colleague telling me that he would describe my clinical work as "secular theology." This comment perturbed me for some time. He elaborated and suggested what he believed to be the most powerful aspect of my clinical work was what occurred between clients, family members, and myself—what he called the phenomena of "reverencing." I pondered this observation for some time and reflected on the meaning of reverence. I have come to believe that "reverencing" is when there is a profound awe and respect, mingled with love, for the individuals seated in front of me. I often feel that same reverencing from clients and family members returned to me.

In those moments of reverencing in clinical work, something very special happens between the healthcare professional and the individual or family; it is something felt by all—a deep emotional connection. I know and have felt these moments in clinical work, whether directly in the room with the family or from behind a one-way mirror as a supervisor or team member. During these times, I have witnessed the most profound changes in family members' thinking, behavior, illness experience, and, most importantly, in their suffering. In these instances, I have felt an emotion that seems to arise only when there is reverencing. This emotion I submit is pure love. To illustrate the power of love in our therapeutic conversations, I wrote/produced an educational DVD in India with two women (a sister and sister-in-law) that beautifully illustrates how the power of love has the potential for healing and softening illness suffering (Wright, 2016).

But, what kind of love? The kind of love that I am referring to is love that opens space to the existence of another beside us in daily living (Maturana & Varela, 1992). But, what does it mean to "open space" to another? It means to be open to their particular ideas, opinions, or beliefs. And, here is the most important aspect, while suspending all judgment.

As healthcare professionals, it means suspending all judgment about our patients'/families' illness experience, their illness suffering, and their choices for illness healing/treatment options. It is what I prefer to call "curious compassion."

The more curious we are about a patient/family's illness suffering, the more we can dissolve our own judgments and biases and practice in a space of curious compassion. It is in this space that opportunities can arise for healing, that loving interactions can flourish. This is the kind of love to strive for in one's clinical practice with individuals/families.

I have come to understand and recognize moments of reverencing and love as one dimension or aspect of the spiritual nature of my clinical work with families that perhaps invites colleagues and students to comment that they observe a "spiritual" aspect to my work with families.

In my personal life, I observed and was amazed by the way my mother coped with adversity with such courage, patience, graciousness, and an incredible non-complaining attitude. She had the capacity, even amidst a horrible, debilitating illness and chronic pain, to experience joy out of small pleasures such as watching the birds out her window or enjoying watching hockey games on television with my father. Here was a vibrant and enthusiastic woman, who worked until she was seventy-two years old, now confined to one room.

She constantly expressed her appreciation and gratefulness for all that was done to care for her. I learned from my mother that deep suffering has the potential to refine and enabled other qualities of her character to shine through. We were frequently amazed as a family how on many days, even when she could no longer walk or feed herself, we would ask, "How was your day?" to which she would respond, "I have had a wonderful day."

A wonderful day? How could she have a wonderful day not being able to get out of bed on her own, brush her hair, walk, feed herself, or even scratch her nose? I needed to understand more, so one day I asked, "Mom, what keeps you going?" and she said, "The love of my family, especially your father. He is so good to me! I just hope that I will not become too much of a burden for my family or that they will tire of visiting me." I continue to be amazed and in awe both personally and professionally of the power of love. When illness robs you of all your faculties and dignity, love still sustains your spirit.

Challenging Constraining Beliefs about Illness Suffering

Our own beliefs as healthcare professionals can hinder or enhance the possibilities for softening suffering (Wright & Bell, 2009). One belief frequently offered to those suffering with illness is that "life could be worse." This belief is benevolently offered to provide comfort and encouragement. One woman, suffering from irritable bowel syndrome, did not find this belief useful. She responded, "I know life could be worse. I could have only one eye or leg, and I am very fortunate to have all I do have... But, those comments do not cure my disease, do not get rid of the pain, the tears, the frustrations, or the losses that come with this condition." This example highlights the need for healthcare professionals to recognize that each person's suffering with illness is unique and that attempting to have persons "count their blessings" can inadvertently trivialize deep suffering. Often persons who are spared from dying by a life-threatening illness or accident find that their lives and relationships are dramatically altered and changed. They are often given direct and indirect messages by well-meaning healthcare professionals that they should be thankful and grateful that things were not worse. "At least you are here." We, as healthcare professionals, need to challenge such beliefs and recognize that we cannot judge what should make life meaningful and purposeful for another. But, rather, we need to assist others to embrace life and find meaning and purpose that is meaningful to them.

Brain science offers explanations that connect how certain family interventions that soften suffering and challenge constraining illness beliefs may result in changes in brain structure and functioning (Wright, 2015). Softening suffering has the additional benefit of calming the amygdala. The amygdala has obtained recent infamy as a panic button of the brain. The amygdala is activated by both positive and negative emotional experiences, but this activation is unequal; it registers negative/fearful experiences more than positive/pleasant ones. The two small, almond-shaped structures known as the amygdala are located in the temporal lobe, also considered to be part of the limbic system. These small groups of nuclei perform a powerful function in memory processing and emotional reactions.

Suffering can trigger the amygdala into a stress response of negative and discouraging beliefs about an illness experience because the amygdala is prepared to activate in response to fearful or potentially threatening inputs (Arden & Linford, 2009). Dealing with serious illness is certainly a life experience that can trigger the amygdala into a fearful response. If healthcare professionals can calm the amygdala, it results in more positive and hopeful beliefs about an illness. Despite families experiencing great suffering and despair in their relationship with illness, by assisting them to rewire their brains, we can help them achieve a calmness and positivity that invites resilience and courage. Learning how to be calm means less suffering, less anxiety, less fear, and less hopelessness. One of the most powerful ways to calm the amygdala is by challenging constraining illness beliefs.

Constraining beliefs invite and deepen suffering.

CLINICAL PRACTICE EXAMPLE: "WILL I EVER BE WHOLE AGAIN?"

I now offer a detailed therapeutic narrative with some of the verbatim therapeutic conversations between the clinician and a loving and courageous couple, Bill and Myrna, fifty-one and forty-seven years respectively, and our clinical team at the Family Nursing Unit, University of Calgary. This therapeutic narrative highlights how conversations about suffering and spirituality can be brought forth, explored, invited, and distinguished, to hopefully invoke healing. This couple was referred to our outpatient clinic by their family physician. One of our Masters of Nursing students, Juliet Thornton (JT), who was the clinician with this family. Other members of the clinical team consisted of graduate nursing students, and two faculty supervisors, of which one was myself! In total, we had five sessions with this couple, and their two adult sons also attended two of the sessions. At the time of referral, Bill was experiencing the aftermath of a stroke and was in remission with leukemia. Sadly, Bill's stroke occurred during his chemotherapy treatment for his leukemia. He was noticeably affected by this stroke with a number of neurological deficits, including some difficulty with speech, cognition, and left-sided weakness in both his arm and leg.

Bill was no longer able to teach in the public-school system, which he had enjoyed so much for twenty-seven years.

In the first meeting with individuals or families, we make it a routine practice to ask the 'one question question' (Wright, 1989; Duhamel, Dupuis, & Wright, 2009). Specifically, "If there was just one question that you could have answered during our work together, what would that one question be?" By asking this question, I believe that we are often able to identify the area of greatest suffering. Frequently, this is *not* the particular presenting concern. The responses to this question I believe come from a different place, and a deeper place within a person than is answered by the question "what is your greatest concern?" Of course, the question "what is your greatest concern" is also a useful question for identifying potential emotional or spiritual suffering and one that suits more the beginning stages of a meeting. The 'one question question,' we have learned in our practice, seems more fitting to be asked towards the end of a first meeting with an individual or family members once a beginning therapeutic relationship has begun.

It became apparent that Bill had many questions about his future that were causing deep suffering due to such losses at the young age of fifty-one years and compounded by no apparent answers that brought relief or meaning. One of the questions that was uppermost in his mind was wondering if his physical progress had progressed as far as it would and, therefore, should he accept it or would there be further recovery? Healthcare professionals, understandably, were reluctant to give any definitive answers to this aspect of his recovery. But, this 'not knowing' sunk Bill into a place of hopelessness, depression, and weeping. Myrna fell into the interactional trap that many spouses, and yes healthcare professionals too, often stumble upon—what I refer to as the "cheer-up phenomena." The more a loved one or client shows sadness or discouragement, the more cheering up and encouraging is done. Frequently, these well-intended acts of kindness to "cheer up another" only enhance one's suffering rather than diminish it because the person does not have their suffering validated, but rather it is walked over, ignored, or minimized. Myrna also wondered what the future held for her husband and queried her role in this dilemma of 'pushing or not pushing;' encouraging or not encouraging her husband to do more. In the therapeutic dialogue that follows, notice how quickly we learn of the impact and influence of this illness upon all family members. Illness and the suffering that is embedded within it, is indeed a family affair!

First Session

Myrna: Like, do we just wait? Do we wait for Bill to get out of that space or should I be pushing him?

Should he be trying more—is it normal to do what he's doing or should we be pushing him more? Or should we not push him and just leave him the way that he is? This is really affecting our family. It's hard for both of us and for our sons. You never realize the difference.

Bill: It is catastrophic...

Myrna: Yeah. Like people think that he's so lucky that he's come through and he's done so well. And, he has. But, it changes your whole life.

Bill: Yeah...

Myrna: Like I'll say to him 'it could be worse you know' but that doesn't seem to help. Because you know it could be a lot worse. Maybe he wouldn't be walking or talking or anything else. But, that doesn't help him. He just has a lot of trouble dealing with what he has left.

Bill: I don't know whether you can provide me with strategies, um, how do you get a person to accept the way they are? I don't know whether that's just something I'm going to have to work on. Maybe I'm going too fast. Maybe I expect too much. I don't know.

JT: So, what I'm hearing now, and this can change as we work together, is that you would like some advice on how to live in this space that you're experiencing right now.

Myrna: Yeah. Are we doing the right thing or the wrong thing?

JT: OK

Myrna: Is it, like I don't know. Sometimes, I think I want to push him and I want to shake him and say, at least you're here. And, other times, I understand it's so hard for him. It's fine to say well at least you can still walk, but the fact that he can't use his arm and his speech is impaired—I guess in terms of, am I doing the right thing? Should I just leave him alone. But, when I try to do that I feel that's wrong. I should be encouraging him.

JT: And, so your hope really is to find some strategies to learn to live with Bill's condition?

Bill: Yeah. Like I don't know what the future is going to hold and that really bothers me because—what is going to happen? Like, am I just going to continue this way throughout my life, like just veg? Or what am I going to do? I just—I don't know.

Myrna: Like when he gets really—like he will sit and cry. "What's to become of me?" And, that breaks my heart when I hear him like that. I felt that way when he was sick and I thought is this going to be our life, you know? It's scary. Nobody thought he would come this far, but will it ever come all the way back? When do you give up and accept that 'this is as good as it gets?' You never give up. But, nobody gives any answers.

JT: And, what do you (looking at Bill) think about Myrna's thoughts about what the future holds?

Bill: Yeah, I agree with her. I don't know whether I should get pushed more. Half of me says I should be thankful and just take each day as it comes, but when you're used to having a life and I don't have much of a life. It just seems more and more (weeping) has been taken away from me—my teaching, my driver's license; it just keeps adding up. So, I don't know whether to try or I don't know whether to give up. Am I beating myself against a wall (weeping)? Should I accept the way it is? But, I don't want to accept that.

Comment/Reflections: Indeed, life has lost all meaning for Bill. It is now a life of contradictions, dilemmas, and great suffering. The poignancy of his suffering is almost palpable even on the pages of this text. His deep suffering is magnified as his beliefs are challenged and altered as exemplified by his comment: "half of me says that I should be thankful... but I don't have much of a life." The numerous losses Bill has experienced impede his ability to be grateful for his life as it invites him to think about what has been lost and, therefore, what IS the purpose of his life now? This lack of purpose and meaning for his life connects his suffering to issues of spirituality. The conceptualization of the Trinity Model is readily apparent and useful here as Bill's illness beliefs, suffering, and spirituality are so closely intertwined! This is now where illness beliefs, suffering, and spirituality begin to connect.

Second Session

In the second session, the illness suffering around Bill's condition emerged again. But, it is incredibly difficult to listen to stories of illness suffering. However, I harbor a profound belief that talking is healing, particularly talking about stories of suffering from illness. I also believe that this healing occurs not just in the emotional domain, but also in the physical domain. Many, many individuals and families over the years have shared how their physical symptoms have diminished or disappeared when they experienced softened suffering. When suffering is softened, it can also result in distinct physiological changes (Wright, 2015).

I also believe that Bill needs to be able to fully tell his illness narrative without being interrupted, cheered up, or stopped in his storytelling. Knowing that this would be a difficult task for our young clinician Juliet, I made a supervisory phone-in (intercom phone-in system between myself as supervisor and the clinician) to offer some direction and support to the student. I pointed out the interactional pattern between Bill's suffering and Myrna's attempts to cheer him up. Every time Bill expressed any verbal or non-verbal suffering, Myrna would interrupt by attempting to cheer him up and Bill would then become silent and suffer more internally, which in turn invited Myrna to continue her efforts to cheer him up and thus the cycle continued. I asked this young, compassionate clinician to just listen to Bill's story, without interruption, without further questions, without any immediate reflection. Juliet beautifully implemented this phone-in and even took it a step further by requesting, most gently of Myrna, that

Suffering and Spirituality

BOTH she and Juliet would "just listen" to Bill. This was a very different experience for both Myrna and Bill. Bill's speaking is preceded by almost a minute of silence and deep, deep sighing on his part. This is a prelude to allowing his illness suffering to come forward, and come forward it did.

JT: I guess I would just like to invite both of us, myself and you, Myrna, to kind of sit back and let you (*Bill*) talk about your situation and what you're thinking. So, if that's okay, we'll just be quiet and listen and then you can tell us when we can talk.

Myrna: You just say what you feel.

[Bill sighs several times and there was a long period of silence. Neither the clinician nor Myrna spoke. Then, Bill begins his tale of suffering.]

Bill: Some days I just feel—well, it is really hard—it is hard accepting the way things are. I tell myself that I should, that I should be thankful that I'm alive, that these things have happened to me and I have to accept them, but I just get really frustrated that I cannot do things like I used to. I trip over things. I understand that my brain doesn't work the way it used to *(silence).* I sit on my balcony and I see people walking and riding and walking their dogs without looking like a gimp and I am a gimp *(sobbing).* I don't know what I'm going to do. I think a lot about that. I can't take each day as it comes and live life being thankful that I didn't die. I have Myrna here with me. But, so much is unknown. I know it sounds silly cause there is always the unknown, but at least like Myrna knows she's going to work, she's got her job—she's got this, she's got that. I <u>don't</u> know. And, you know, you come here (referring to Juliet) and talk to us and things like that. You've got some sort of schedule to your life. Like my doctor said she'd die to have two weeks off. I, uh, I do not know what my future is going to hold and I think a lot about that. Maybe I should not, I don't know. (Pause) If I could do something beneficial. I just do not want to spend my time getting up, making the bed, doing the dishes, doing the laundry. Like I don't mind doing that, it is not like I hate it. But, there has got to be something more. And, it is just coming to accept that. I guess it is going to take—well, I know it is going to take time. But, I just uh... *(sighing)* Am I making any sense?

JT: Yes. Is it okay, Bill, if we talk?

Bill: Sure.

JT: Okay. I am just wondering what you (Myrna) are thinking as you listen?

Myrna: I just feel his pain and I know that he—if you could have known what he was like before his illness and how just the kind of person that he is, you would realize how difficult this is for him. And, I just can feel his pain. And, I feel so helpless because—but when he is like this at home we can talk about it, but sometimes he won't talk. It is just the same thing, but I do not understand, I do not know what to do. When he gets like this—I know what he is going through in a sense because I feel it—we are a part of each other and just like he feels my pain, I feel his. And, I hate leaving him some days. And I come home at lunchtime and he cries and it takes everything I have to go back to work. It takes everything I have. And, these little jaunts where I take a couple of days off—like I went back to work Jan. 24th and I have not taken a sick day since I returned to work cause I was off from June until January. When I get overtired or for vacation or whatever I used to have these extra days off with him so that we can do things. Even things as mundane as doing chores, but it is together.

Comments: At this point, I again call Juliet on the intercom system and offer a couple of suggestions for questions that could be asked. Juliet then shares my questions with the couple.

JT: The team just had a couple of questions. They are just wondering if you believe that talking is healing for you?

Bill: Yes and no. I look forward to these sessions. It's good to talk. It's good to get the feelings out. Cause if I am just with Myrna I know that I don't always talk. But, um, I do not (crying), I don't see any future for me.

Myrna: You described it as a vicious circle.

Bill: Yes, it is a vicious circle and I go around and around and around cause I do not see any end near. Cause sometimes I think this is what my whole life is going to be. Right now, I do not see answers. People haven't got answers for me. Like, I don't know, maybe I am rushing too much. I am off (work) until the beginning of

January and then I'll see the doctor. Um, I'm anxious to get going on doing something. I have got to feel that there is some meaning to my life. I don't know. The other day I was thinking about the kids—about teaching, about my classroom. That is not there for me anymore. Cause I know I won't be able to go back teaching, but (sighing) there's got to be something more. I don't know. It's a vicious circle.

Comments/Reflections: Talking is healing! But, it is not any rambling, undirected talking. It is talking that has occurred when a healing context has been created, when reverencing has occurred between Juliet, Bill, and Myrna and when the illness story has been invited in a particular kind of way that enables healing to begin. The telling of this illness narrative with all its embedded suffering was the *first* time that Bill had been invited to relate his story of suffering and strength. This was a pivotal and profound moment in the therapeutic sessions. A space was created for Bill's suffering to come forth by the manner in which Juliet and Myrna listened to his story without judgment, without a need to respond, without further questions, and without attempts to cheer him up. It is this kind of listening and witnessing that creates the possibility for healing to occur. But, what a gift for all!

At the end of each session at the FNU, the family was offered the opportunity to listen to the ideas and reflections of our clinical nursing team. If they desired to hear the team, then we asked if there were any questions they had for the team or that they would like the team to address. We referred to this process as the Reflecting Team (Anderson, 1987). Then, the clinical team would come into the interviewing room and the family would go behind the one-way mirror to listen and observe, and have their own reflections while the team was discussing their situation. The one question that Bill wanted the team to consider was, "Will I ever be whole again?" Whereas Myrna's question was, "Are we heading down the right path? Is there anything else out there that can help?" The following is part of the verbatim discussion during the Reflecting Team. The clinical team consisted of graduate nursing students, Dr. Janice M Bell (JMB), and myself (LMW) as faculty supervisors.

Reflecting Team Discussion

LMW: So, do we feel brave enough to tackle this very difficult question they are asking? So, Bill was asking, 'Will I be whole again?' and earlier he was asking should I be accepting—was that the question? 'Should I be accepting this or should I be pushing myself more?' That seems like a dilemma throughout the whole interview, wasn't it? And, then, for Myrna it was 'Are we heading down the right path?' Did she have a question earlier?

JT: Well, advice—she was wondering about advice for

how to live in this space she called it.

LMW: I mean one of the things they are saying is that nobody can tell them? They're saying they want to know, is this as far as I can go? Or can I go further?

JMB: Or should I push myself?

LMW: Or should I push myself further? And, I guess I would like to not give them the party line again today and say we don't know how you're going to progress. I am willing to step out on a limb. And, I would like to say that I think he *can* go further. That I think he *should* push himself. Because I think not pushing himself is not healthy for him right now. He does not feel good about that. I think he should push himself and test his limits to see what he is capable of. Instead of waiting for the health professionals to say 'yes, you are going to get better' or 'you are not.' No. Let him discover.

JMB: Well, it sounds like they have had lots of really interesting experiences already of challenging healthcare professional beliefs about even whether Bill was going to live.

LMW: Yes. Health professionals try to be responsible and say prepare yourself on one hand (for a shortened life), but miracles happen—if they think of this as a miracle. So, I am saying now he has survived, for what purpose and for how far he can go, I do not know that. But, I do know—I do believe very strongly that he should push himself. That he should push beyond and not wait for an answer from someone else. That he should decide his own limits. And, another thing that I want to offer them I learned from a woman who was a quadriplegic who was in a terrible car accident. She was a psychologist and taught a workshop that I went to. And, she taught me something that's been very useful to me in my work with families. She said that you never—when health professionals are suggesting you should accept this—she said you never have to accept it. You never have to accept what has happened to you. But, you do have to adjust to it. And, I think that is a wonderful distinction. Bill may never want to accept that he does not have the full use of his right hand. That he maybe has some memory problems from time to time. That his right leg does not work as it once did. He never has to fully accept that. But, he *does* have to adjust to it. That is what I'm saying. But, adjust to what? He does not know the limits yet because he is waiting for somebody to give him direction about how far to go. And, I am saying push the limits. Go for it. See how far you can go.

JMB: I take it that you think the uncertainty about that invites inertia in him.

LMW: Yes, it invites inertia and I think it invites his depression. I think it invites him to feel very emotional wondering 'Is this as good as it gets or is it not?' Should he accept it or should he not? I am saying he does not have to accept it. It is a terrible thing that has happened to him. It is a tragedy. He is right, at fifty-one years old. And, so, my answer I guess to Myrna's question is the same. When she is asking 'Should I be encouraging, should I be pushing him?' I say push him. Get in there and let us see what he is capable of. And, no more of this sitting around and trying to figure out 'should we just sit here and accept it or should we not?' I mean, I just think this man has got a lot to offer. I do not know where he will end up finding himself. Maybe he will end up being at home on his computer doing interesting things—writing. Maybe he will want to get a part-time job. Maybe he will want to get full-time work somewhere. I do not know, but I think he will not know that until he pushes more. But, I am curious about the rest of you (asking other team members). What do you think? Do you perhaps disagree with what I am saying? Is there another way to look at that?

Nursing Student: I get the impression that he is already starting to push himself. Just doing all the work at home. I mean all the courage it takes for a man to accept or adjust to that. To do it and to learn to do the cooking like Myrna was mentioning. I think it is another way to push himself. Because it was probably not something that he was very pleased about at the beginning, but now he is doing it. And, also, like Myrna was mentioning, now he is going to the computer, even though she is worried that he is spending all his time on the computer looking for answers. I think it is another way to push.

LMW: Yes, that is true.

Nursing Student: She even mentioned that the time that he is at the computer his attention is there. He feels better looking for more answers, but, at some point, maybe he will say okay I can see then that I cannot get an answer or he is going to get an answer that is going to fit for him and he will push himself a bit more. But, for me, what I saw today I really had the impression that both of them are already pushing.

LMW: You are right. Maybe he has already started.

JT: Well, I think he is very determined and creative.

Comments: I took a very strong position in offering my own beliefs about what might be helpful for Bill. Was it a useful position to take? The proof is in the pudding. Immediately after the team's discussion, the family is invited back into the interviewing room and the team returns to its position behind the one-way mirror. Now, the viewing angles are shifted once again, as the team now listens to the family's reflections on the team's reflections. We encourage the clinician to now ask the family, "What stood out for you?" as a means of knowing of all the ideas that were offered, which of the ideas "fit" with the person's biopsychosocial-spiritual structure (Maturana & Varela, 1992). In other words, which comments, opinions, or offerings by the team invited a reflection in that particular person. Change that occurs through reflection, we have learned in our clinical practice, provides the most sustaining and powerful change. "The moment of reflection… is the moment when we become aware of that part of ourselves which we cannot see in any other way" (Maturana & Varela, 1992, p. 23). A reflection can be about the past, present, or future. It does not just mean looking back. Reflections on the present and future can be powerful influences as well.

Bill's response to my suggestion to "push the limits" was one of the comments he reported to Juliet (following the team's discussion) that he found most useful. For Bill, this was his most significant reflection. Other questions could have also invited a reflection such as, "If you never push yourself, what do you predict your life will be like in six months?" or "Do you think being in a dilemma about pushing yourself adds or diminishes stress on your body?" In addition to questions, we can invite others to a reflection by offering ideas, advice, and suggestions that can serve as useful perturbations (Wright & Levac, 1992). Of course, most healthcare professionals work independently and do not have the benefit of a reflecting team, but learning how to ask reflective questions, and offering our best professional knowledge through advice and opinions can be equally as useful. It is only when healthcare professionals are invested in the outcome (i.e. expecting someone to follow our advice or believing our opinion is the correct one) that there is a likelihood that minimal or no change will occur. With invitations to reflection, the challenging of constraining beliefs that invite suffering commences. Bill was suffering dreadfully with his constraining belief that perhaps he should just accept what had happened to him. By inviting Bill and Myrna to a reflection, the "truth" of their stance, which was a constrained solution (not pushing himself), was challenged. It was then possible to offer, entice, and invite them to a differing belief that may have the possibility of reducing suffering and giving his life more meaning (Wright & Bell, 2009). We cannot *make* people believe something different. We cannot *give* them a new facilitating belief. It happens through the process of mutual reverencing between the healthcare professional and client/family and invitations to reflection.

This family has graciously given me permission to utilize the therapeutic narratives in written publications, professional conferences, and research. They participated in McLeod's (2003) hermeneutic inquiry to explore the meaning of spirituality and spiritual care practices in family systems nursing. In a research interview with Dr. Deborah McLeod some two years after our clinical work was completed, they again reported that the most useful aspect of their five sessions at the FNU was the advice to "push the limits" (McLeod, 2003). Myrna also commented on her experience with the team at the Family Nursing Unit (FNU) in being invited to "push the limits." Myrna found herself seeking spiritual answers. She attributed this seeking to the listening and questioning of the team. Part of this very revealing, informative, and helpful research interview following the completion of our clinical work with this couple, which occurred with Dr. Deborah McLeod (DM), is offered below

(McLeod, 2003, p. 168).

DM: So, it was the idea of pushing the limits that you both found the most helpful?

Myrna: Yes, pushing the limits was the biggest thing, but also looking inside yourself for the answers.

DM: Can you tell me a little bit about that?

Myrna: Well instead of looking to the outside for answers, they encouraged us to look to the inside.

DM: Can you say something about how they did that?

Myrna: Well, when we discussed our spiritual beliefs, they supported those and they followed through and asked more questions, which made you think more about your own beliefs. Their beliefs didn't come into it. They didn't try to direct you towards their beliefs or any other beliefs. They listened to what you believed. They accepted that and supported it and questioned it to bring it out more, which makes you think about it more.

Bill: We definitely did more thinking about it.

Myrna: Yeah. The fact that they brought our beliefs into the discussion and that they found our beliefs interesting and that they were accepting of it, you know. That made me more comfortable to be able to talk about it. I was surprised at how they wanted to discuss that aspect of our lives.

Comments: Previously, Bill and Myrna had refused visits from clergy, believing (rightly or wrongly) that such persons are associated with particular systems of religious beliefs that would not be congruent with their own beliefs. However, their experience at the Family Nursing Unit was experienced differently as they claimed being heard allowed for a deepening and strengthening of their beliefs without being directed to believe in a particular way, which would have enhanced their suffering.

Sadly, at the time of the research interviews, Bill was experiencing a recurrence of leukemia and a bone marrow transplant. Myrna offered her insight during the research interviews that having the opportunity to speak about their faith beliefs made a positive difference in how they were dealing with their latest health crisis.

Myrna: They (the nurses at the FNU) were prepared to listen to something that doesn't fit into a specific category of formal religion. And, that support made a big difference for us and for the kids. We were really thankful for the sessions and we just kept growing spiritually since then. Until the wheels all fell off in May, when the leukemia came back. But, I think the fact that we were there and we had those sessions helped us to deal with it better this time.

These powerful, reflective comments by Myrna are not only tremendously gratifying to us a clinical team, but also indicate how changes can continue to reverberate for some time and be useful when further illness challenges or crises occur. As too often happens, this family had not previously met any healthcare professionals who had an interest in their illness suffering or in their spiritual beliefs about their suffering, even though they had experienced two previous life-threatening situations.

Healthcare professionals missed the privilege of hearing and learning from Bill and Myrna about their current spiritual beliefs. "Bill and Myrna believed that all experience, including experiences of suffering, occurred for the purpose of learning. It seemed, however, that Bill's suffering was influenced in part because these beliefs were inadequate to address his experience for now. He seemed to hold this belief intellectually, but not in his heart. Myrna, however, found these beliefs to contain much hope for her and she believed that if Bill would simply remember and hold onto this belief, if only he would look for the learning contained in this present experience, his suffering would be eased" (McLeod, 2003).

Each individual has numerous beliefs operating and emerging every day, about every situation and every person encountered. But, not all beliefs matter; not all beliefs invite an emotional or physiological response (Wright & Bell, 2009). The beliefs that do matter are our core beliefs. We all possess core beliefs, which are personal and often unconscious. Core beliefs are fundamental to how we approach the world; they are the basic concepts by which we live. Our core beliefs are our identity and are accompanied by intense affective and physiological responses. Core beliefs are the "beliefs that matter" within our relationships and within significant events in our lives, such as illness.

Therefore, when differences arise between family members around their core beliefs, particularly in the midst of much suffering and a life-threatening illness, it adds additional suffering and strain, even in the best of relationships such as Bill and Myrna's. For example, Bill "no longer found the belief that there was learning in his suffering of any comfort. His struggle to reinterpret this belief provoked strong feelings and fear for Myrna, yet her fear was not that he had no belief that was comforting exactly. Her thought was that *if only* Bill would find spiritual meaning in his current situation, Myrna could let go of some of the fear that she was holding for Bill" (McLeod, 2003). Bringing forth Bill and Myrna's suffering about the illness and its dramatic aftermath through particular and skillful questioning, triggered new reflections about the illness and their lives.

This particular case example hopefully provides the reader with another illustration of the conceptualization and usefulness of the Trinity Model (see Chapter 4). The example also illustrates the application of several of the spiritual care practices highlighted in this chapter.

The clinical work with this courageous and loving family was most rewarding and gratifying. Both Bill and Myrna's suffering was dramatically softened through many emotional, cognitive, and behavioral changes that occurred during the therapeutic process. They regained their hope for their future and Bill was able to once again find meaning and purpose to his life. Also, powerful healing conversations, facilitated by Juliet, occurred between the parents and their sons as preferences for future illness crises were clarified. But, this positive and effective clinical work could not have taken place without the reverencing, love, and compassion that occurred between Bill, Myrna, and Juliet. As their therapeutic relationship unfolded in each session, their profound respect and awe deepened for one another. The evidence for the reverencing in their relationship was the numerous conversations of affirmation and affection that were brought forth in each meeting (Wright & Bell, 2009). Plus, the clinical team also had a special affection for this family and the family for them, reverencing and love had occurred!

It is with sadness that I also must tell of the passing of Bill from a recurrence of his leukemia and bone marrow transplant two years after our clinical work at the FNU. We are very grateful and indebted to this family for their generosity of spirit in so willingly giving their permission to share our clinical work with them. It is hoped that their story will provide healthcare professionals with new ideas for their practice with individuals and families. In so doing, I trust that I have honored Bill's contribution to our and my learning as a clinical team and the legacy to his family in a manner that is respectful and loving. Of course, the names of this family were changed for reasons of confidentiality, but their spirits that shine through on the pages of this text are not anonymous.

Concluding Thoughts

For those healthcare professionals who choose to work where deep suffering is frequently or routinely encountered, I hope that the spiritual care practices offered in this chapter will supplement their current knowledge, caring, and competence with patients/families. However, can all healthcare professionals offer spiritual care practices in their work with individuals and families? Perhaps not. Perhaps there is some self-selection of healthcare professionals who choose to work in areas where more often deep suffering occurs such as emergency units, oncology units, palliative care, long-term care, hospice and/or caring for the wounded and injured in times of war or natural disasters. Healthcare professionals are quite aware that deep suffering, dying, and grieving are an integral part of these particular practice areas. But, even then, some professionals may simply choose, consciously or unconsciously, not to practice in areas where deep suffering is prominent or front and center. But, this is not to judge one healthcare professional as being more valued than another. It is best when we practice where there is the best fit of our competencies, knowledge, and passion. And, certainly, there is work enough for all.

REFERENCES

Andersen, T. (1987). The reflecting team: Dialogue and meta-dialogue in clinical work. *Family Process, 26,* 415-428.

Arden, J. B., & Linford, L. (2009). *Brain-based therapy with adults: Evidence-based treatment for everyday practice.* Hoboken, NJ: John Wiley.

Bell, J.M. (2016). The central importance of therapeutic conversations in family nursing: Can talking be healing? *Journal of Family Nursing 22(4),* 439–449 doi: 10.1177/1074840716680837.

Dossey, B.M. (2000). *Florence Nightingale: Mystic, Visionary, Healer.* Springhouse, PA: Springhouse Corporation.

Duhamel, F., Dupuis, F., Wright, L.M. (2009). Families' and nurses' responses to the "One Question Question": Reflections for clinical practice, education, and research in family nursing. *Journal of Family Nursing, 15*(4), 461-485. doi:10.1177/1074840709350606.

Frank, A. (2013). *The wounded storyteller: Body, illness and ethics. 2nd Ed.* Chicago: The University of Chicago Press.

Houger Limacher, L., & Wright, L.M. (2006). Exploring the therapeutic family intervention of Commendations: Insights from research. *Journal of Family Nursing, 12,* 307-331. doi:10.1177/1074840706291696.

Maturana, H.R., & Varela, F.G. (1992). *The tree of knowledge: The biological roots of human understanding* (Rev. Ed.). Boston: Shambhala.

McLeod, D.L. (2003). Opening space for the spiritual: Therapeutic conversations with families living with serious illness. Unpublished doctoral thesis, University of Calgary, Alberta, Canada. (Supervisor: Dr. Lorraine M. Wright) Retrieved from http://dspace.ucalgary.ca/handle/1880/45183.

Walsh, F. (2016). Applying a family resilience framework in training, practice, and research: Mastering the art of the possible. *Family Process,* 55, 616-632.

Wright, L. M. (2015a). Brain science and illness beliefs: An unexpected explanation of the healing power of therapeutic conversations and the family interventions that matter. Journal of Family Nursing, 21, 186-205. doi:10.1177/1074840715575822.

Wright, L.M. (2015b). Eckhart Tolle's spiritual words of wisdom: Application to family nursing practice. *Journal of Family Nursing* 21(4) 503–507. doi: 10.1177/1074840715606244.

Wright, L.M. [Producer]. (2007). *Spirituality, Suffering, and Illness: Conversations for healing.* [DVD]. (Available from: www.lorrainewright.com/sufferingdvd.htm).

Wright, L.M. (Producer). (2016). *Therapeutic Conversations with Families: What's love got to do with it?* [DVD]. (Available from: www.lorrainewright.com/lovedvd.htm).

Wright, L.M., & Bell, J.M. (2009). *Beliefs and illness: A model for healing.* Calgary, AB: 4th Floor Press.

Wright, L.M., & Leahey, M. (2013) 6th Ed. *Nurses and families: A guide to family assessment and intervention.* Philadelphia: FA Davis Co.

The Path to Illness Healing

Sections of this chapter have been reprinted with permission from "Spirituality, Suffering, and Beliefs: The Soul of Healing with Families" by L.M. Wright (2009) in Froma Walsh (2nd Ed.) *Spiritual Resources in Family Therapy.* New York: Guilford Press

Chapter 6

Connecting the Personal and the Professional

Suffering and joy teach us, if we allow them, how to make the leap of empathy, which transports us into the soul and heart of another person. In those transparent moments we know other people's joys and sorrows, and we care about their concerns as if they were our own.
Fritz Williams

If you have been reading this book from the first page, I hope it is now obvious that we must connect, integrate, and acknowledge our personal and professional lives in matters of suffering and spirituality. This is imperative in order to bring forth more genuine and useful therapeutic conversations with patients and families. Of course, there will be differences in our abilities due to age and life experiences. Some healthcare professionals are young in years, others may be inexperienced in matters of suffering, or perhaps their spiritual beliefs are different or less well developed than their patients. Even if there does exist some shortcomings in life experience, or of a healthcare professional's own spiritual development, they can still be enormously helpful to patients and their families in their encounter of suffering. Being compassionate and caring can be accomplished if healthcare professionals will embrace being a particular kind of healthcare professional, one who possesses curious compassion, love, and non-judgmentalness about illness suffering and healing. In addition, we need an overarching theoretical model for practice, such as the Trinity Model, to inform and guide our practice (see Chapter 4); and having specific spiritual care practices that mark the path to illness healing (see Chapter 5). All of these suggestions and ideas will help, in addition to our own learning of how to be vigilant and cognizant about the reciprocity between our personal and professional lives with regards to suffering and spirituality (Wright, 1997).

PERSONAL TO PROFESSIONAL

How do we connect our personal experiences to our professional lives in ways that can bring forth greater compassion and understanding for those who suffer serious illness? One such experience helped me profoundly to understand the phenomena of 'living in a different world' than those who live daily with serious illness, disability, or loss.

Just one year into my mother's ordeal, I wrote an email to a close friend and entitled it, DAMN MS. 'Just got off the phone from my parents and, yes, my mother is having another MS attack. They are going to try and avoid another hospitalization and give her steroids on an outpatient basis, but it will depend on how the next few days go… her legs are numb tonight and the pain is terrible. I must say that my spirits have been knocked, my dad sounded knocked also. My poor mom! What a damn illness! Is this what it's going to be like from now on…?? I sensed that my mom is trying to be brave, my dad sounds defeated. Well, I think I'll make some mint tea and try and soothe my spirits."

I am impressed and struck by my use of the word "spirit" to describe the effect of my suffering. Spirit and suffering were now connected in my personal life, as well as my professional life.

Surprisingly to me, I did not experience that it was onerous at that particular time, when surrounded by others who were suffering, either personally or professionally. Rather, it was comforting to be in the presence of others whose lives were also engulfed in suffering. There seemed to be an unspoken bond amongst us who were suffering, simply by the way we were experiencing our world. My suffering seemed to even be enhanced and difficult in the presence of others whom I judged, unfairly I admit, were too frivolous, too superficial, too concerned with life's trivia, or even too happy. But, they were simply living their lives, experiencing joy, as we all do when suffering has not caught our attention for a time, or, worse yet, consumed us. Yes, those who suffer do live in a different world from those who are living their fortunate lives without deep suffering!

PROFESSIONAL TO PERSONAL

Frequently, we do not recognize or give credit to the numerous times our caring for patients and families bring great benefits to our own personal lives and relationships. We can be under the illusion that we are doing all the 'giving,' and hopefully healing, by diminishing or softening suffering in our caring for patients/families. We may not recognize that the stories of suffering, strength, compassion, endurance, and love that we hear and witness in the midst of serious illness, are offering us hope, inspiration, and even guidance for our own lives. Clinical practice is certainly not a one-way street of offerings where we give our best professional knowledge, opinions, and compassion, but, rather, the patients and families with whom we meet are also changing and benefiting our lives, perhaps more than we are aware or care to acknowledge.

One such example for me was a young man who was diagnosed with MS. When I met him, he was just in his early thirties and experiencing great emotional suffering from his condition. During my meeting with him and his parents, I inquired, "What's the toughest part about managing MS every day and coping with it?" This therapeutic conversation was not about symptoms, or medication, or treatment, but rather about this young man's illness experience; the specific intention was to understand the potential or actual areas of suffering. He gave a poignant response, "Things that seemed so trivial, I can't really do anymore. They're not really important things, but everyone does them."

This young man helped me to learn and remember that many of the daily tasks and routines that are normally out of our awareness and taken for granted are gone **out** of his capabilities and **into** his awareness in the context of illness. I was reminded of my own personal experience in assisting my mother with bathing, dressing, and eating. Turning on the water taps, doing up your own brassiere, and spreading jam on your toast are just a few of the things that, as this young man taught me, "are not really important things, but everybody does them." That is, everybody but this young man, my mother, when living, and countless others for whom these tasks and routines accentuate their dependence on and difference from others (Wright & Bell, 2009). Serious illness often disrupts taken-for-granted ways of being in the world. Such disruptions often lead to suffering, and therefore can trigger a search for meaning. This one example of my own learning I have often passed on and transferred to other patients and families with whom I have worked. I now fully appreciate that the inability to do everyday tasks becomes everyday pinpricks of the constant and unrelenting reminders to those who have a serious illness or disability that their lives have substantially, and often irreversibly, changed. My best learnings always come from the patients/families themselves, supplemented by the professional literature and my own and others' research.

Our Life Experience is Not our Patient's Life Experience

Often, there is a tendency and temptation among healthcare providers to offer their own understandings, their own "better" or "best" meanings or beliefs for their clients' suffering experiences with serious illness. For example, one family related to me that following their son's death from a motor vehicle accident, a nurse suggested, "It must be your son's time, otherwise he would not have died so young." But, these supposedly well meaning comments were not comforting to this family. It did not decrease their deep suffering. As the family related, "Maybe that was this nurse's explanation or understanding, but it was not ours. We are still searching for a satisfying explanation for our son's death." One way to avoid this trap of prematurely offering explanations or advice to soften suffering is to remain insatiably curious about how clients and their families are managing in the midst of suffering. And, especially, what they believe about their illness experiences or loss and what meaning they give to their suffering (Wright & Bell, 2009).

Being insatiably curious, coupled with compassion, can be one of the most rewarding, enlightening, and educating experiences for healthcare professionals, both personally and professionally (Wright, 2015). How **do** those who suffer with serious illness make sense of their lives? How are their family members responding and reacting? What have they found helps them to cope? What influence, if any, do their spiritual or religious beliefs have on their suffering?

Healthcare professionals who possess curious compassion put on the armor of prevention against blame, judgment, or the need to be "right." Asking therapeutic or reflexive questions (Tomm, 1987; Wright & Bell, 2009; Wright & Leahey, 2013) invites a person to explore and reflect on their **own** meanings of their suffering, not the healthcare professional's. Hopefully, in those reflections of our therapeutic conversations we have with our patients/families, healing may be triggered as new thoughts, ideas, or solutions come forth, are pondered and considered about how to best live one's life with illness.

Inviting reflections happens through very deliberate and thoughtful questions. Examples of questions that I have found very useful to invite curious compassion (Wright, 2015a) are:

- *What questions do you find yourself asking these days (about your illness or your suffering)?*
- *Have you come to any understanding about your suffering?*
- *How do you make sense of your suffering?*
- *What parts of your suffering are hardest to make sense of? What's that like for you?*

Of course, we also learn from families for future clinical work and our own relationships. Therefore, there are questions we need to pose to ourselves about the influence of our clinical work.

- *What will I take away or have learned from this patient/family that will benefit me in future work with other families?*
- *What will I take away or have learned that will help me in my personal life?*
- *What will I never forget about this patient/family?*
- *What belief(s) of mine was challenged or confirmed through my clinical work with this individual or family? (Wright & Bell,*

2009).

In my own life and in the lives of those whom I have cared for, I have experienced that, after a time, some of the stories and meanings of suffering lose their usefulness and there is a need for new conversations that yield fresh meanings, that "renarratize" or bring hope.

After one particularly difficult visit to my mother, I found myself unable to watch or participate in her emaciated, quadriplegic body being turned one more time by her lovely and compassionate caregivers. As I walked down the hallway from her room, feeling the salty tears on my cheeks, I became aware of a conversation that I was having with myself. "What more can I learn from my mom's suffering? I have nothing more to learn. I cannot watch her suffering nor understand it anymore." The previous stories of why my mother suffered, of why I and my family suffered and what might be learned from it that had been so useful in the past, had now worn thin! I needed a new story, a new meaning, a new ray of hope. When meaning-making breaks down, our explanatory conversations and their particular meanings lose their vitality, and thus we often find suffering, conflict, or alienation are not far behind.

So, what does help in these moments? I have found the words of a Rabbi written in ca. 930 to be most profound and consistent with my own beliefs. He said, "Comfort the sufferer by the promise of healing, even when you are not confident, for thus you may assist his natural powers" (Israeli, Manhig HaRofiem). Yes, as healthcare professionals we need to offer the promise of healing and hope to the very end! We need to assist our patients in finding the kind of hope that is meaningful for **them**. Of course, this does not necessarily mean the kind of hope that someone will be cured of illness, or their loss reversed, but rather the hope that they will find meaning to their suffering, that they will know that their life is still important and cherished in the lives of others and, most importantly, to themselves, despite the changes their illness has brought to their life and to their most intimate relationships.

LEARNING AND OFFERING THROUGH COMMENDATIONS

Commendations tend to highlight individual and family members' strengths, competencies, and resources (Houger Limacher, 2003; Houger Limacher & Wright, 2006; Wright & Leahey, 2013; and Wright & Bell, 2009). In a fluent and moving piece of research conducted by Houger Limacher (2003), she focused specifically on the intervention of commendations as offered in the clinical practice at the Family Nursing Unit, University of Calgary. A key to uncovering was both families and nurses reported and reiterated the value and power of commendations that brought forth 'goodness,' and helped soften their suffering (Houger Limacher, 2003). This bringing forth of "goodness" becomes a relational phenomena in the context of the nurse-patient/family relationship. Commendations have the power to create and bring forth 'goodness,' or what I refer to as 'particular kinds of persons' who possess a 'particular way of being in the world.' This particular kind of person, and way of being in clinical practice, is someone who looks for strengths amidst suffering, hope amidst despair, and meaning amidst confusion. "We become our conversations and we generate the conversations that we become" (Maturana & Varela, 1992). These types of therapeutic conversations entered into by healthcare professionals who bring forth 'goodness' are what I believe form the structure and foundation of spiritual practices. This way of being in the world connects and integrates our personal lives to our professional lives and vice versa.

SPIRIT MATTERS

When we soften or diminish suffering within our therapeutic conversations with patients/families, we are touching or reawakening dampened, discouraged, and distraught spirits. Illness, and often the suffering experiences that accompany illness, can demoralize and oppress lives, relationships, and our very spirits. I believe the more that we are able to connect suffering and spirituality in our professional and personal lives, the more we, as individuals, will be well integrated and well equipped to succor and support those who suffer. Yes, spirit matters.

IN CLOSING

How does one end a book on spirituality, suffering, and illness? However, this book may be described or named, my sincere hope is that within its pages we have all been invited and called, myself included, to further reflections about suffering, spirituality, illness, hope and healing. Hopefully, healthcare professionals reading this book have gleaned some new understandings and ideas for inviting and listening to conversations about suffering and spirituality with patients and their families so opportunities for healing may begin. It is hoped that the Trinity Model (Chapter 4) and the Spiritual Care Practices (Chapter 5) will be new additions for your clinical practice. And, of course, all the knowledge and healing occurs within and between the relationships of the 'trinity' of patient, family, and healthcare providers.

Under the blows of mortal experience, those who suffer from serious illness, loss, or disability need reassurance, comfort, hope, love, and, above all, the knowledge and reassurance that they are still cherished. This kind of practice is indeed spiritual and one that offers a great opportunity and blessing for all healthcare professionals.

REFERENCES

Houger Limacher, L. (2003). *Commendations: The healing potential of one family systems nursing intervention.* Unpublished Doctoral thesis: University of Calgary.

Houger Limacher, L., & Wright, L.M. (2006). Exploring the therapeutic family intervention of Commendations: Insights from research. *Journal of Family Nursing*, 12, 307-331. doi:10.1177/1074840706291696.

Tomm, K. (1987). Interventive interviewing: Part II. Reflexive questioning as a means to enable self-healing. *Family Process*, 26(6), 167-183.

Wright, L.M. (1997). Multiple sclerosis, beliefs and families: Professional and personal stories of suffering and strength. In S. McDaniel, J. Hepworth, W.J. Doherty (Eds.), *The shared experience of illness: Stories of patients, families, and their therapists* (pp. 263-273). New York: Basic Books.

Wright, L.M. & Leahey, M. (2013) *6th ed. Nurses and families: A guide to family assessment and intervention.* Philadelphia: FA Davis Co.

Wright, L.M., & Bell, J.M. (2009). *Beliefs and Illness: A Model for Healing.* Calgary, AB: 4th Floor Press.

MOVIES THAT ADDRESS ILLNESS SUFFERING AND/OR LOSS

Here is a list of a few of my favorite movies that offer poignant stories of illness suffering, loss, hope and healing. The list includes movies that focus on physical and mental, life-shortening and chronic illness. Some of the movies illustrate the impact of illness on family relationships and reciprocally the influence of family relationships on illness. A few of the movies also deal with issues of spirituality and religion.

STILL ALICE (2014)

A linguistics professor and her family find their bonds tested when she is diagnosed with Alzheimer's Disease.

Koffler, P.; Lutzus, L.; Brown, J.(Producers) & Glatzer, R. & Westmoreland, W. (Directors). (2014). USA: Killer Films.

THE THEORY OF EVERYTHING (2014)

An in-depth look at the relationship between the famous physicist Stephen Hawking, who suffers with Lou Gehrig's disease, and his wife.

Bevan, T.; Fellner, E.; Bruce, L.; & McCarten, A. (Producers) & Marsh, J. (Director). (2014). UK & USA: Working Title Films Ltd.

AUGUST: OSAGE COUNTY (2013)

Family relationships are portrayed in this deeply moving movie in which words are used as weapons. The impact of illness, suicide, secrets, substance abuse.

Clooney, G.; Heslov, G.; Doumanian, J.; Traxler, S. (Producers)
& Wells, J. (Director). (2013). USA: Jean Doumanian
Productions; Smokehouse Pictures; Battle Mountain Films; &
Yucaipa Films.

AMOUR (2012)

The narrative focuses on an elderly couple, Anne and Georges, who are retired music teachers with a daughter who lives abroad. Anne suffers a stroke which paralyses her on the right side of her body.

Haneke, M.; Menegoz, M.; Arndt, S.; Heiduschka, V.; Katz, M.
(Producers) & Haneke, M. (Director). (2012). *Amour* [motion
picture]. France: Sony Pictures Classics.

DEPARTURES (2008)

A Japanese movie with English subtitles of a devoted cellist who becomes unemployed and finds new work preparing bodies for burial. Although his wife is disgusted by the work he begins to perfect the art of "Nokanshi," a profound journey with death as he uncovers the wonder, joy and meaning of life and living.

Mase, Y., Nakazawa, T., Nobukuni, I., Watai, T. (Producers) &

Takita, Y. (Director). (2008). *Departures*. Japan: Amuse Soft Entertainment.

THE DIVING BELL AND THE BUTTERFLY (2007)

The true story of Elle editor Jean-Dominique Bauby who suffers a stroke and has to live with an almost totally paralyzed body; only his left eye isn't paralyzed.

Kennedy, K. & Kilik, J. (Producers) & Schnabel, J. (Director). (2007). France: Canal+Kennedy/Marshall Company & France 3 Cinéma.

AWAY FROM HER (2006)

A man coping with the institutionalization of his wife because of Alzheimer's disease faces an epiphany when she transfers her affections to another man.

Egoyan, A., Hirst, V., Iron, D., Mankoff, D., Urdl, S., Weiss, J. (Producers) & Polley, S. (Director). (2006). *Away from Her*. Canada, UK & USA: The Film Farm & Foundry Films.

A BEAUTIFUL MIND (2001)

After a brilliant but asocial mathematician accepts secret work in cryptography, his life takes a turn to the nightmarish, a story of schizophrenia.

Grazer, B., & Howard, R. (Producers) & Howard, R. (Director). (2001). US: Imagine Entertainment.

Iris (2001)

True story of the lifelong romance between novelist Iris Murdoch and her husband John Bayley, from their student days through her battle with Alzheimer's disease.

Dreyer, M., East, G., Fox, R., Hedley, T., Minghella, A., Pollack, S., Rudin, S., Thompson, D., Weinstein, H. (Producers) & Eyre, R. (Director). (2001). *Iris*. Uk & USA: British Broadcasting Corporation (BBC), Fox Iris Productions, Intermedia Films, Mirage Enterprises & Miramax Films.

Philadelphia (1993)

When a man with AIDS is fired by a conservative law firm because of his condition, he hires a homophobic small time lawyer as the only willing advocate for a wrongful dismissal suit.

Demme, J. & Saxon, E. (Producers) & Demme, J. (Director). (1993). US: Clinica Estetico.

Shadowlands (1993)

A 1993 British biographical film about the relationship between English academic C. S. Lewis and American poet Joy Davidman, her death from cancer, and how this challenged Lewis's Christian faith.

Attenborough, R., Clegg, T., Eastman, B., Hawkins, D., Webb, A. (Producers) & Attenborough, R. (Director). (1993). *Shadowlands* [motion picture]. UK: Price Entertainment.

About the Author

Lorraine M. Wright, RN, PhD, completed her doctoral studies in marriage and family therapy and has been a practicing marriage and family consultant/therapist for over forty years. Her expertise in family relationships has extended to couples and families suffering with serious illness by combining her original discipline of nursing with marriage and family therapy. Dr. Wright is also an international speaker, author, and blogger. She is also a Professor Emeritus of Nursing, University of Calgary, Canada, where for twenty years she directed an outpatient clinic, the Family Nursing Unit, for couples/ families suffering with serious illness.

In addition, she has written/co-written fifteen professional books; numerous book chapters and articles; and produced/co-produced ten educational DVDs.

Dr. Wright has received several honours and awards for her distinguished contributions and leadership in family nursing and family therapy from the American Association for Marriage and Family Therapy, the American Family Therapy Academy, and the International Family Nursing Conference. Dr. Wright has received two honorary doctorates from the University of Montreal, Canada, 2008, and Linnaeus University, Kalmar, Sweden,

2012. In 2013, she was awarded a Queen Elizabeth II Diamond Jubilee Medal in Canada. She is a much sought-after speaker and has offered keynotes, lectures, workshops, and consultations in over thirty countries.

Her goal is to visit 100 countries to learn about healthcare professional practices' that relieve and soften illness suffering. To that end, Dr Wright has now visited 70 countries.

AUTHOR CONTACT INFORMATION

Lorraine M. Wright, RN, PhD

Email: lmwright@ucalgary.ca
Blog: www.lorrainewright.com/blog
Twitter: @drlorwright
Websites:
www.lorrainewright.com
www.FamilyNursingResources.com
www.IllnessBeliefsModel.com

Available for keynote addresses, lectures, and/or workshops related to the following topics:

• Suffering and Spirituality: The Path to Illness Healing

• Illness Beliefs of Patients/Families and Healthcare professionals: The Greatest Influence to Healing

• Therapeutic Conversations: What's Love Got to do with it?

• Don't Get Married...Unless: Why Most of Us are not Marriage Candidates and What to do About It

Index

accepting what is   *29, 33, 35*
affiliation   *25, 93, 102, 103, 110, 113. See also religion*
   church affiliation   *102*
alleviation of suffering. *See also religion*
amygdala   *32, 198*
appeal of complementary, integrative, or alternative healing approaches   *187*
attendance. *See also religion*
   church attendance   *110*
attention to suffering   *36, 53*
   lack of attention to suffering   *36*

beliefs
   about illness   *10, 30, 129, 160*
   constraining   *10, 30, 33, 44, 74, 129, 156, 160, 186, 215*
   core   *128, 129, 219, 220*
   facilitating   *74, 86, 129, 141, 142, 156, 171*
   family systems   *61, 63, 78, 102, 119, 216, 239*

care, spiritual   *2, 7, 8, 10, 55, 64, 87, 89, 92, 94, 96, 101, 106, 107, 108, 109, 112, 115, 116, 119, 145, 158, 159, 160, 161, 175, 216, 220, 222, 228*
cheer-up phenomena   *201*
chronic pain   *20, 21, 23, 35, 45, 54, 143, 182, 183, 195*
church affiliation. *See also religion*
   and attendance   *102*
commendations   *48, 63, 64, 78, 153, 165, 171, 190, 191, 192, 236, 237*
   commendations to the family   *153*
constraining beliefs   *10, 30, 33, 44, 74, 129, 156, 160, 186, 196, 215*
conversations, therapeutic   *2, 10, 26, 27, 37, 39, 46, 54, 57, 59, 60, 61, 62, 63, 64, 65, 66, 73, 81, 92, 100, 105, 106, 108, 115, 121, 123, 144, 156, 158, 159, 166, 175, 193, 194, 199, 223,*

224, 227, 233, 237
core beliefs   *128, 129, 219, 220*
curiosity   *84, 108, 152, 167, 168*
   maintaining   *108*
curious compassion   *100, 165, 195, 228, 233, 234*

deep suffering   *1, 2, 5, 14, 15, 18, 19, 20, 22, 23, 24, 26, 35, 36, 39, 42, 43, 44, 45, 46, 55, 56, 58, 69, 71, 83, 84, 85, 99, 106, 107, 115, 116, 160, 172, 176, 178, 181, 196, 197, 200, 204, 222, 223, 230, 232*
despair   *32, 198, 237*
distress   *18, 23, 35, 51, 84, 86, 110, 115, 143, 145*
distress, spiritual   *18*

emotional   *21, 23, 35, 36, 49, 57, 60, 87, 97, 135, 142, 143, 155, 176, 194, 198, 200, 205, 212, 219, 221, 230*
   and/or spiritual suffering   *49, 142, 155, 176, 200*
   and physical suffering   *135*
   connection   *194*
   domain   *205*
   reactions   *198*
   suffering   *230*
   symptoms   *87*
empathy   *95, 173, 174, 227*
engaging   *10, 44, 63, 105, 123, 160*
   in therapeutic conversations   *105*
   suffering strangers   *10, 160, 166*
everyday life   *13, 20, 23, 25, 35, 39, 56, 143*. See also *religion* See also *experience*
   changes in   *39*
   forced exclusion from   *23, 35, 55, 143*
experience. See also *everyday life*;
   connect our personal experiences to our professional lives   *228*

facilitating beliefs   *74, 86, 129, 141, 142, 156, 171*

about life *86*
and commendations *171*
constraining beliefs versus *129*
that soften suffering *74*

family
experiences *49, 129*
interventions *27, 64, 121, 186, 197, 224*
spirituality *97, 98, 103*
support *63, 80, 186*

Family Nursing Unit (University of Calgary) *vi, x, 60, 65, 77, 78, 108, 130, 157, 187, 199, 216, 218, 236, 244*
commendations as offered in the clinical practice at the *236*
outpatient clinic of the *x*

family spirituality *98, 103*

fear *42, 71, 105, 147, 148, 156, 172, 181, 198, 220*
learning to live without *181*
of dying *147, 148*
the most common *147*

FNU. *See also Family Nursing Unit (University of Calgary)*

goodness *64, 237*
embedded in commendations *64*

healing *i, ii, 1, 4, 5, 6, 7, 11, 35, 57, 90, 116, 130, 157, 181, 182, 225, 239, 246*
conversations *221*
facilitating *2*
opportunities for *238*
power of love *8, 101*
promise of *236*
talking is *26, 174, 209*

health outcomes *101, 103, 110*

hermeneutic *62, 63, 64, 65, 66, 80, 109, 216*
research *63, 80*

hope *x, 2, 3, 8, 11, 15, 38, 44, 45, 60, 72, 73, 74, 75, 76, 77, 104, 105, 107, 109, 116, 124, 136, 152, 154, 158, 159, 175, 176, 178, 184, 186, 187, 196, 203, 219, 221, 222, 227, 230, 235,*

    236, 237, 238, 240
    and illness healing   *2*
    Illness stories of   *44*
    the genesis of   *38*

illness. *See illness narrative*
    beliefs about   *10, 30, 129, 160, 196*
    constraining beliefs about   *196*
    healing   *i, ii, 1, 2, 4, 11, 12, 40, 54, 85, 86, 87, 92, 100, 195, 228, 246*
    narrative   *15, 33, 37, 39, 40, 44, 47, 53, 74, 79, 189, 205, 209*
    relational effect of   *46*
    research specifically addressing   *65*
    stories   *x, 9, 25, 39, 44, 45, 57, 85, 99, 144, 175*
Illness Beliefs Model   *6, 61*
illness diagnosis   *46, 47, 189*
illness narrative   *15, 33, 37, 39, 40, 44, 47, 53, 74, 79, 189, 205, 209*
illness narrative(s)   *ix, 14, 20, 22, 23, 26, 39, 175, 176. See also suffering, stories of*
illness stories. *See also illness narrative(s)*
interconnectedness   *11*
    of beliefs, suffering, and spirituality   *11, 157*
intervention research, to soften suffering   *60*
interventive questions   *47*
inviting reflections   *233*
    about illness suffering   *10, 160, 186*

judgment   *84, 100, 164, 194, 195, 209, 233*
    suspending all   *84, 100, 194, 195*
    trust, compassion, and understanding without   *164*

karma   *93*

learning   *6, 7, 60, 87, 145, 162, 166, 168, 181, 188, 191, 215, 219, 220, 222, 228, 231*

The Path to Illness Healing

letters, therapeutic   63, 79
life experiences. *See also everyday life*
listening   10, 57, 58, 74, 78, 99, 108, 144, 160, 171, 174, 175, 176, 177, 209, 216, 238
   deep   171, 177
   to, and witnessing stories of illness suffering   174
   to conversations about suffering   238
   to illness stories   57, 144
love   vii, 1, 7, 8, 12, 17, 23, 35, 38, 48, 52, 56, 72, 85, 99, 100, 101, 105, 118, 143, 155, 156, 164, 165, 173, 175, 187, 190, 191, 192, 194, 195, 196, 221, 224, 228, 230, 238
   and compassion   7
   between and among family members and therapists   38
   spiritual care practices that have a foundation of   7
   the healing power of   8, 101

meaning-making   97, 235
medical narrative   37
medical perspective   51

needs, spiritual   101, 105, 106, 108, 113, 186
Nightingale, Florence   94, 95, 117, 121, 158, 159, 223
nurse (s). *See also nursing*
   nursing. *See also nursing*
   open space to spirituality   108
   perceptions of spirituality and spiritual care practices   107
   therapeutic conversations between nurses and families   62, 81, 108
   therapeutic letters written by   63
nursing   vi, 7, 11, 14, 27, 58, 60, 63, 67, 77, 78, 79, 80, 81, 89, 90, 94, 95, 96, 101, 102, 106, 110, 115, 119, 120, 121, 146, 154, 159, 174, 199, 209, 210, 216, 223, 224, 239, 244. *See also nurse (s)*
   history of spirituality in   94
   research   101
   responsibility for spiritual care   96
   spirituality in   4, 7, 8, 9, 10, 11, 13, 20, 88, 90, 94, 96, 102,

104, 106, 116, 120, 145, 238

objectification of spirituality   *114, 161*

pain, chronic   *20, 21, 23, 35, 45, 54, 143, 182, 183, 195*
patients. *See also family*
    and families   *33, 53, 113, 128, 129, 130, 143, 161, 185, 186, 227, 230, 232*
    spiritual or religious beliefs   *86, 87, 103, 112, 233*
    therapeutic conversations with   *10, 26, 39, 46, 61, 106, 108, 123, 227, 237*
pedagogy of suffering   *55, 117*
personal experience   *ii, 90, 172, 231*
prayer   *98, 107, 180*
professional literature. *See also research*

reflection, inviting. *See also research*
religion   *5, 6, 8, 9, 13, 25, 30, 37, 41, 85, 88, 89, 90, 92, 96, 101, 102, 103, 110, 111, 112, 113, 115, 117, 118, 119, 128, 147, 167, 218, 240*
    definition of   *25, 92*
    distinction between spirituality and   *25*
research
    intervention research to soften suffering   *60*
    specifically addressing illness suffering in therapeutic conversations   *65*
reverencing   *10, 38, 85, 155, 156, 160, 177, 193, 194, 195, 209, 216, 221*

self   *22, 43, 50, 98, 105, 148, 186, 191, 222, 239*
self-selection   *222*
self-soothing   *50*
softening suffering   *3, 10, 36, 57, 66, 186, 196, 230*
soul   *13, 17, 18, 19, 24, 29, 44, 66, 67, 81, 83, 84, 91, 93, 99, 121, 156, 227*
soul care   *99*

spirit. *See also spirituality*
spiritual care   *v, 158, 160, 238*
   practice   *8, 101, 161*
spiritual distress   *18, 145*
spirituality
   family   *97*
   objectification of   *114, 161*
   research about   *102*
spiritual needs   *101, 105, 106, 108, 113, 186*
suffering   *10*
   acknowledgment of   *172*
   alleviation of   *143*
   concept in the Trinity Model   *143*
   definition of   *77*
   diminishing   *33*
   illness and   *63, 105*
   medical perspective   *51*
   resisting   *31*
   softening   *3, 10, 35, 36, 57, 66, 186, 196, 230*
   spiritual   *36, 49, 57, 60, 86, 135, 142, 143, 176, 200*
   stories of. *See also illness narrative(s)*
   trivialize   *54*
suffering and spirituality   *ix, 1, 2, 3, 4, 7, 8, 9, 10, 12, 13, 20, 23, 26, 27, 54, 199, 227, 228, 238*
suffering, stories of   *x, 13, 21, 38, 64, 82, 85, 121, 175, 176, 205, 230, 239*
sympathy   *95*

talking is healing   *26, 72, 144, 174, 205, 208, 209*
therapeutic conversations   *vii, 2, 8, 10, 12, 26, 27, 37, 39, 46, 54, 57, 59, 60, 61, 62, 63, 64, 65, 66, 73, 81, 92, 100, 101, 105, 106, 108, 115, 121, 123, 144, 156, 158, 159, 166, 175, 193, 194, 199, 223, 224, 227, 233, 237, 246*
   about illness suffering   *37, 73, 92*
   research specifically addressing illness suffering in   *65*
   with healthcare professionals   *26*
   with patients/families   *46, 106, 237*

therapeutic letters   63, 79
Tolle, Eckhart   29, 31, 35, 39, 40, 43, 81, 121, 224
transformation   34, 84, 85
Trinity Model   v, 10, 11, 27, 55, 61, 123, 124, 125, 126, 130, 143, 144, 156, 204, 220, 228, 238
   Beliefs Concept in   126
   Spirituality Concept in   144
   Suffering Concept in   143

University of Calgary, Family Nursing Unit   x, 77, 130, 199, 236
unspeakable, speak the   72, 133, 141

witnessing   10, 38, 54, 58, 85, 99, 144, 160, 174, 175, 176, 179, 184, 209
   illness stories   85, 175
   suffering   10, 54, 160

www.ingramcontent.com/pod-product-compliance
Lightning Source LLC
Chambersburg PA
CBHW071000160426
43193CB00012B/1859